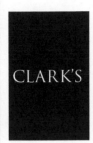

CLARK'S

ESSENTIAL GUIDE TO

CLINICAL ULTRASOUND

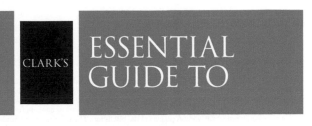

ESSENTIAL GUIDE TO

CLARK'S

CLINICAL ULTRASOUND

Jan Dodgeon
Former Senior Lecturer and Programme Leader
University of Salford, UK
Associate Professor
Oslo Metropolitan University, Norway

Gill Harrison
Professional Officer for Ultrasound
Society and College of Radiographers
London, UK

Series Editor for Clark's Companion Essential Guides:

A Stewart Whitley
ISRRT Director of Professional Practice & Radiology Advisor
UK Radiology Advisory Services
Preston, Lancashire, UK

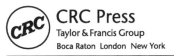

CRC Press
Taylor & Francis Group
Boca Raton London New York

CRC Press is an imprint of the
Taylor & Francis Group, an **informa** business

First edition published 2023
by CRC Press
6000 Broken Sound Parkway NW, Suite 300, Boca Raton, FL 33487-2742

and by CRC Press
4 Park Square, Milton Park, Abingdon, Oxon, OX14 4RN

CRC Press *is an imprint of Taylor & Francis Group, LLC*

© 2023 Jan Dodgeon and Gill Harrison

ISBN: 9780367775087 (hbk)
ISBN: 9780367771164 (pbk)
ISBN: 9781003171706 (ebk)

DOI: 10.1201/ 9781003171706

Typeset in Linotype Berling LT Std
by Evolution Design & Digital

CONTENTS

Foreword   ix
Preface   xi
Acknowledgements   xv
Abbreviations   xix

Chapter 1 Principles of sonography   1

Overview of diagnostic ultrasound   2
Patient preparation and care   21
Safety considerations   26
References   34

Chapter 2 The upper abdominal organs   39

The pancreas   43
The liver and biliary system   48
The portal venous system   55
The spleen   58
References   63

Chapter 3 The renal tract   67

The kidneys   68
The urinary bladder   78
References   84

Chapter 4 The male reproductive system   87

Transrectal ultrasound (TRUS) of the prostate gland   88
The scrotum and testes   92
The penis   103
References   105

Contents

Chapter 5 The gastrointestinal (GI) tract 107

The salivary glands   108
The adult GI tract   112
Endoscopic ultrasound (EUS)   117
The neonatal GI tract   121
References   124

Chapter 6 The endocrine system – thyroid and adrenal glands 127

The thyroid gland   128
The adrenal glands   135
References   139

Chapter 7 The female reproductive system 141

Gynaecological ultrasound   142
Hysterosalpingo-contrast sonography (HyCoSy)   152
Assisted reproduction   157
References   161

Chapter 8 Obstetric ultrasound 165

Overview   166
Early pregnancy assessment   169
First trimester   175
Second trimester   179
Third trimester   188
References   194

Chapter 9 Breast ultrasound 197

Greyscale, Doppler and contrast-enhanced ultrasound (CEUS)   198
Elastography   204
Volume scanning   206
References   209

Chapter 10 The cardiovascular system 211

The aorta 212
The extracranial arterial supply to the brain 217
Peripheral arterial – lower limb 223
Peripheral arterial – upper limb 230
Peripheral venous – lower limb 232
Peripheral venous – upper limb 237
Echocardiography 239
Transoesophageal echocardiography 249
Intravascular ultrasound 252
References 255

Chapter 11 The respiratory system – lungs 257

The lungs 258
References 265

Chapter 12 The central nervous system – eye and brain 267

Ocular ultrasound 268
The neonatal brain 272
References 278

Chapter 13 Musculoskeletal ultrasound 279

The shoulder 280
The elbow 285
The wrist and hand 289
The paediatric hip joint 294
The knee 303
The ankle and foot 308
Ultrasound-guided interventions 314
References 318

Contents

Chapter 14 Emergency and interventional ultrasound 321

Emergency ultrasound: FAST   322
Interventional ultrasound   330
References   335

Chapter 15 Additional technologies 337

Contrast-enhanced ultrasound (CEUS)   338
Fusion imaging   341
Artificial intelligence (AI) in ultrasound   344
References   349

Index   351

FOREWORD

It has been a delight to witness the development and publication of *Clark's Essential Guide to Clinical Ultrasound*. This latest addition to the *Clark's* series of pocket and desktop books is a testament to the skills, knowledge and dedication of the authors who are key members of the radiography profession and who have at heart the desire to share their knowledge and experience with sonographers at the start of their career and those who seek to further their knowledge.

Miss K C Clark, I am sure, would welcome this important addition to the series which has its origins in the recently published *Clark's Procedures in Diagnostic Imaging (A System-Based Approach)* which included the use of ultrasound in the diagnosis of many diseases and conditions. This book, however, is dedicated specifically to the use of sonography and will be a valuable aid and resource for the diagnostic/medical ultrasound, radiography and healthcare communities.

This book conveys to its readers an immense amount of important knowledge that is current and relevant and essential to modern-day sonographic practice.

The patient must surely benefit by this publication.

A Stewart Whitley
Series Editor
ISRRT Director of Professional Practice &
Radiology Advisor
UK Radiology Advisory Services
Preston, Lancashire, UK

PREFACE

This *Essential Guide to Clinical Ultrasound* is part of the *Clark's* series of diagnostic imaging books. This particular title aims to provide an overview and guide to a wide range of ultrasound examinations.

Every patient's journey into healthcare must start with a diagnosis, and almost every diagnostic pathway includes imaging. Add this to the fact that ultrasound is the most widely used modality in the world after plain radiography, and the importance of ultrasound becomes clear. The figures in England alone bear this out,[1] showing that there are more ultrasound examinations performed than CT and MRI scans combined. In those parts of the world where more expensive equipment is beyond reach, the proportionate use of ultrasound is even higher, and its importance in medical care and diagnosis even more crucial.

This expanding use of ultrasound has led to technical advances and an ever-increasing range of applications, creating a demand for accessible information on the best use of ultrasound in diagnosis and interventions. This textbook, covering the essentials of ultrasound, will be of help both to learners and to practitioners who are asked to scan an area beyond their usual practice, or who encounter advances in technology for the first time. While many users will reach for the internet to expand their knowledge, a printed book sets information in context, enabling the reader to re-read and cross-reference more easily than when scrolling on a screen. Research has shown that readers of print books absorb and remember more information than readers of e-books do, and that students who read texts in print scored significantly better on the reading comprehension test than students who read the texts digitally.[2] Purchasers of this book can have the best of both worlds, with access to the printed version for depth of information and overall context, and an e-version for quick and easy reference in the clinical setting. As ultrasound is a highly skilled, dynamic examination, this textbook aims to assist the reader to develop the appropriate underpinning knowledge, but cannot replace the need for supervised hands-on clinical practice, experience, assessment of clinical skills and continual audit of clinical practice.

Of course, there are already many ultrasound textbooks available, but as lecturer-practitioners and ultrasound programme directors, the authors have often struggled to find textbooks that are at the right level for students and also cover the range of topics that are required for today's practice. We have written this book to this end, acknowledging that in today's healthcare setting it is not enough for sonographers to capture a series of images; they must also analyse what they see before them in real time, interpret findings, determine whether to extend the examination, and write clear, comprehensive, actionable clinical reports, and recommend further management options, if applicable. We have therefore used the highest available standards to suggest a comprehensive imaging procedure for each examination.

The operator dependence of this dynamic imaging modality raises the bar for competency and continuing education, and the underlying science for this is outlined in the first chapter, 'Principles of sonography'. There follow 12 chapters based on anatomical systems, each including a short introduction, indications for referrals, patient preparation, the imaging procedure, and finally an image analysis section covering the more common findings. Each chapter has a full reference list. The last two chapters cover generic applications in emergency and interventional ultrasound, and the use of new technologies – contrast imaging, fusion imaging, and artificial intelligence.

We have sought out the latest research for this book, and the timing of the COVID-19 pandemic has enabled us to include some of the latest ultrasound diagnostics for this. However, it could be noted that some of our references may be a few years old – but we would argue that these are not necessarily out of date. After all, nobody would refute Christian Doppler's paper 'Concerning the coloured light of double stars', which contained the first statement of what we now describe as the Doppler effect, just because it was published in 1842. Thus, we have on occasion referenced an original source of research, rather than a more recent secondary review that quotes a previous publication merely in the interest of having the latest date on the reference. Solid information is a blend of original seminal research and the latest evidence within any specific area; practitioners should continue to supplement their reading with other evidence-based writing and current guidelines as they emerge.

It has been a pleasure to write this book, not least because of the rewarding experience of sharing knowledge with a network of colleagues. It has been a demonstration of the benefits of team working, and we hope we have included all those who have helped in the following acknowledgements.

We close with the old trick question asked of a new recruit: Who is the most important person in the hospital? – the answer, of course, is THE PATIENT. Therefore, we are most grateful of all to those patients who have allowed us to share their images, and who at an often anxious and stressful time, gave their generous consent to enable expansion of all our learning. We must never forget that they are the most important person in all our professional lives.

Jan Dodgeon
Gill Harrison

References

1. NHS England 2021 Diagnostic Imaging Dataset 2021–22 Data. https://www.england.nhs.uk/statistics/statistical-work-areas/diagnostic-imaging dataset/diagnostic-imaging-dataset-2021-22-data.
2. Mangen A, Walgermo BR, Brønnick KK. Reading linear texts on paper versus computer screen: Effects on reading comprehension. *International Journal of Educational Research* 2013;**58**:61–68. doi: 10.1016/j.ijer.2012.12.002.

ACKNOWLEDGEMENTS

We are indebted for the help and advice given by very many colleagues throughout the diagnostic imaging community, with contributions enthusiastically given by sonographers, radiologists, physicists and lecturers from many health institutions, academic departments, the medical imaging industry, professional bodies and special interest groups.

We would particularly like to thank the following individuals for their contributions:

Sue Atkinson, Ultrasound Service Manager, and Debbie Pasquill, Screening Support Sonographer, both of Wrightington, Wigan and Leigh NHS Foundation Trust; Gareth Bolton, Ultrasound Programme Leader, University of Cumbria; Rita Borgen, Consultant Radiographer, East Lancashire NHS Trust; Claire Borrelli, Education & Training Manager, Radiographic Advisor to Public Health England, and Lead Mammographer for England; Helen Brown, Senior Sonographer, and Kashmir Kenyon, Senior Sonographer, both of University Hospitals of Morecambe Bay NHS Foundation Trust; Annette Cox, Senior Sonographer, CARE Fertility, Manchester; Judi Curtis, Mammography Programme Leader, Kingston and St George's, London; Clare Drury, Clinical Specialist Sonographer, Hull University Teaching Hospitals NHS Trust; Lorraine Edwards, Senior Sonographer, and Zoe Mottram, Clinical Lead Sonographer, both of Pennine Acute Hospitals NHS Trust; Dr Ramon Fernando-Alvarez, Consultant Paediatrician, Brighton and Sussex University Hospitals NHS Trust; Erica Henry, Highly Specialised Cardiac Physiologist and Clinical Educator for Adult Echocardiography, Manchester Heart Centre, Manchester Royal Infirmary; Janette Keit, Specialist Sonographer, Blackpool Fylde and Wyre NHS Foundation Trust; Mary Leighton, Senior Sonographer, Lancashire Teaching Hospitals NHS Foundation Trust; Alison McGuinness, Senior Sonographer, Mid Yorkshire Hospitals NHS Trust; Francine Mulenga, Senior Sonographer, Imperial College Healthcare NHS Trust; Dr Sally Norton, Consultant Surgeon, Upper

GI and Bariatric Surgery, North Bristol NHS Trust; Dr Ricardo Ribeiro, Lecturer, Escola Superior de Tecnologia da Saúde de Lisboa, Portugal; Dr S. Sukumar, Consultant Radiologist, Central Manchester University Hospitals NHS Foundation Trust; Anne E Sykes, Lecturer, University of Salford; and Joyce Yates, Consultant Radiographer, Sandwell & West Birmingham NHS Trust, all of whom provided valuable contributions.

In addition, we are grateful for the provision of ultrasound images to: Matt Beardshall, Lead Sonographer, Chesterfield Royal Hospital; Angela Booth, Senior Sonographer, Pennine Acute Hospitals NHS Trust; Hannah Buggey, Vascular Scientist, and Tracey Gall, Senior Clinical Vascular Scientist and Clinical Training Manager, both of Independent Vascular Services Ltd, Manchester; Sophie Cochran, Clinical Specialist in Medical Ultrasound, Pilgrim Hospital, United Lincolnshire Hospitals NHS Trust; Allison Harris, Sonographer, Great Ormond Street Hospital for Children; Simon Hayward, Specialist Physiotherapist, Blackpool Teaching Hospitals NHS Foundation Trust; Dr Abhishek Jain, Radiology Registrar, Central Manchester University Hospitals NHS Foundation Trust; Professor John P McGahan, Department of Radiology, Sacramento, USA; Claire Melia, Sonographer, Northern Care Alliance; Graham Nightingale, illustrator; Nicky Palin, Advanced Clinical Physiologist, Derby Teaching Hospitals NHS Foundation Trust; Pamela Parker, Consultant Sonographer, Hull University Teaching Hospitals NHS Trust; Andrew Picton, Managing Director, Independent Vascular Services Ltd, Manchester; Christine Bunting, Paediatric Sonographer, Central Manchester University Hospitals NHS Foundation Trust; Professor Paul Sidhu, Consultant Radiologist, King's College Hospital, London; Henry Stax, Practical Sonography Facebook site; Kristie Sweeney, Senior Sonographer, Western NSW Local Health District, Australia; Samantha Thomas, Senior Sonographer, Sydney, Australia; Heather Venables, Ultrasound Programme Leader, University of Derby; Lorelei Waring, Senior Lecturer, University of Cumbria, Dr Mike Weston, Consultant Radiologist, St James's University Hospital, Leeds; Patsy Whelehan, Clinical Specialist Radiographer, Ninewells Hospital & Medical School Dundee; Care UK; CIRS (Computerized Imaging Reference Systems, Inc.); NHS FASP and NHS NAAASP.

Finally, thanks are given to the many models who patiently posed for photographs and images. These were mainly radiographers, students and volunteers from a variety of health institutions including the University of Cumbria and the University of Salford, and include:

Joanne Ashworth, Joanne McKenna, Shelly Smart, Lilley Smart, Lorelei Waring and Stewart Whitley.

ABBREVIATIONS

2D	two-dimensional
3D	three-dimensional
4D	four-dimensional
AAA	abdominal aortic aneurysm
ABPI	ankle–brachial pressure index
ABUS	automated breast ultrasound
ABVS	automated breast volume scanning
AC	abdominal circumference
AC joint	acromioclavicular joint
ACR	American College of Radiology
ADNEX	Assessment of Different NEoplasias in the adneXa
AFP	alpha-fetoprotein
AI	artificial intelligence
AIDS	acquired immune deficiency syndrome
AIUM	American Institute of Ultrasound in Medicine
ALARP	as low as reasonably practicable
ALP	alkaline phosphatase
ALT	alanine transaminase
AMV	anterior mitral valve leaflets
AP	anteroposterior
AST	aspartate aminotransferase
AV	arteriovenous
AVM	arteriovenous malformation
AXREM	Association of Healthcare Technology Providers for Imaging, Radiotherapy & Care
BI-RADS	Breast Imaging – Reporting and Data System
BMI	body mass index
B mode	brightness modulated mode
BMUS	British Medical Ultrasound Society
BPH	benign prostatic hypertrophy
BTS	British Thoracic Society
CA125	cancer antigen 125
CASE	Consortium for the Accreditation of Sonographic Education
CBD	common bile duct
CCA	common carotid artery
CEUS	contrast-enhanced ultrasound

Abbreviations

CFA	common femoral artery
cfNIPT	cell-free non-invasive prenatal testing
CFV	common femoral vein
CHD	common hepatic duct
CIRS	Computerized Imaging Reference Systems, Inc.
CMUT	capacitive micromachined ultrasonic transducer
CRL	crown–rump length
CT	computed tomography
CVS	chorionic villus sampling
CW	continuous wave
dB	decibels
DDH	developmental dysplasia of the hip
DHSC	Department of Health and Social Care
DRL	diagnostic reference levels
DVT	deep vein thrombosis
ECA	external carotid artery
ECG	electrocardiogram
ED	erectile dysfunction
eFAST	extended focused assessment with sonography in trauma
eGFR	estimated glomerular filtration rate
EPAU	early pregnancy assessment unit
ERCP	endoscopic retrograde cholangio-pancreatography
ESUR	European Society of Urogenital Radiology
EUS	endoscopic ultrasound
EVAR	endovascular aneurysm repair
FASP	Fetal Anomaly Screening Programme
FAST	focused assessment with sonography in trauma
FGR	fetal growth restriction
FL	femur length
FNA	fine-needle aspiration
FNAC	fine-needle aspiration cytology
FNH	focal nodular hyperplasia
GGT/gamma-GT	gamma-glutamyl transferase
GFR	glomerular filtration rate
GI	gastrointestinal
GIT	gastrointestinal tract
GP	general practitioner
HC	head circumference
hCG	human chorionic gonadotrophin
HCPC	Health and Care Professions Council
HIFU	high-intensity focused ultrasound
HIV	human immunodeficiency virus

HSE	Health and Safety Executive
HSG	hysterosalpingography
HyCoSy	hysterosalpingo-contrast sonography
Hz	hertz (cycles per second)
ICA	internal carotid artery
IOTA	International Ovarian Tumor Analysis
IPEM	Institute of Physics and Engineering in Medicine
IUS	intrauterine system
IVC	inferior vena cava
IVH	intraventricular haemorrhage
IVUS	intravascular ultrasound
kHz	kilohertz (1,000 cycles per second)
LCPD	Legge–Calve–Perthes disease
LFTs	liver function tests
LSV	long saphenous vein
LUTS	lower urinary tract symptoms
MASS	Multicentre Aneurysm Screening Study
MCP	metacarpophalangeal
MHPRA	Medicines and Healthcare Products Regulatory Agency
MHz	megahertz (1 million cycles per second)
MI	mechanical index
ml	millilitres
M mode	movement modulated mode
MRCP	magnetic resonance cholangio-pancreatography
MRI	magnetic resonance imaging
MSK	musculoskeletal
ms^{-1}	metres per second
NAAASP	National Abdominal Aortic Aneurysm Screening Programme
NEC	necrotising enterocolitis
NF	nuchal fold
NHS	National Health Service
NHS BSP	NHS Breast Screening Programme
NHS FASP	NHS Fetal Anomaly Screening Programme
NICE	National Institute of Health and Care Excellence
NIPE	Newborn and Infant Physical Examination
NT	nuchal translucency
OCT	optical coherence tomography
OHSS	ovarian hyperstimulation syndrome
PD	pancreatic duct
PET	positron emission tomography

Abbreviations

PMUT	piezoelectric micromachined ultrasonic transducer
PSA	prostate-specific antigen
PSV	peak systolic velocity
PUJ	pelvi-ureteric junction
PUBS	percutaneous umbilical blood sampling
PV	per vagina
QA	quality assurance
RADS	Reporting and Data Systems
RAS	renal artery stenosis
RCC	renal cell carcinoma
RCOG	Royal College of Obstetricians and Gynaecologists
RCR	Royal College of Radiologists
RI	resistive index
RUQ	right upper quadrant
SCoR	Society and College of Radiographers
SCr	serum creatinine
SFJ	saphenofemoral junction
SMA	superior mesenteric artery
SSV	short saphenous vein
SV	splenic vein
SWE	shear wave elastography
TCC	transitional cell carcinoma
TCD	transcerebellar diameter
TGC	time gain compensation
TI	thermal index
TIA	transient ischaemic attack
TIPSS	transjugular intrahepatic portosystemic shunt
TNM	tumour, node, metastases
TOE	transoesophageal echocardiography
TOS	thoracic outlet syndrome
TQM	total quality management
TRUS	transrectal ultrasound
TVS	transvaginal scan
UKHSA	United Kingdom Health Security Agency
UPJ	utero-pelvic junction
UTIs	urinary tract infections
VA	ventricular atrium
VUR	vesico-ureteric reflux
WRMSD	work-related musculoskeletal disorder
XAI	explainable AI

CHAPTER 1
PRINCIPLES OF SONOGRAPHY

Overview of diagnostic ultrasound   2
Patient preparation and care   21
Safety considerations   26
References   34

OVERVIEW OF DIAGNOSTIC ULTRASOUND

Sonography is the art and science of using ultrasound as a diagnostic modality. Its use as an imaging modality is increasingly popular, and for some years now the sale of ultrasonic imaging devices has outstripped the combined sales of all the X-ray, computed tomography (CT), magnetic resonance imaging (MRI) and nuclear medicine imaging units. There is almost no part of the body for which ultrasound imaging has not been attempted, and so it is essential for today's radiographers and imaging technicians to have some understanding of applications and limitations to ensure the appropriate modality is employed for each condition encountered.

Introduction to the physics of ultrasound

Unlike X-ray energy, ultrasound is not electromagnetic radiation. Ultrasound is very similar to audible sound, although of a much higher frequency. It is a form of energy that travels in waves, propagated by vibration of adjacent molecules in a medium.

The use of ultrasound for imaging is relatively simple technology. A pulse of sound is generated within a transducer – a device that can change one form of energy into another. The sound is transmitted into the body and propagated through the tissues, with gradual attenuation by absorption and reflection. Although some sound is reflected away and scattered, some is reflected back to the transducer as an echo, and this can be plotted on a screen as a dot whose brightness is related to the strength of the returned echo and whose location is calculated by a system known as registration, so that the display replicates the position in the body.

Ultrasonic sound has the same parameters as audible sound, including frequency, speed, wavelength and power.

The frequency of a sound wave is the number of wave fronts that pass a given point per second and is measured in cycles per second or hertz (Hz), or in the case of ultrasound millions of cycles per second or megahertz (MHz). In fact, 'ultrasound' is defined as that which is beyond the range of human hearing, which is about 18 kHz (a frequency of 18,000 cycles per second). Diagnostic ultrasound frequencies are even higher than this, generally in the range of 2–15 MHz.

The speed of sound is constant in a given medium; in other words, the waves travel at a constant speed through a particular medium. This is dependent on the mechanical properties of the medium, principally the density and the elasticity of the substance. Speed is measured in units of distance per unit time, namely ms^{-1}. The speed of sound in formulae is generally represented by 'v' for velocity or 'c' for constant.

The wavelength is the length of a complete wave pattern, or the distance between two successive compressions or two successive expansions. It is measured in units of distance, and represented by the symbol λ, which is the Greek letter L, for length. These three parameters of velocity, frequency and wavelength are linked by the following formula:

$$v = f \times \lambda$$

Because the speed is a constant, there is an inversely proportional relationship between the wavelength and the frequency, so that as one increases the other must decrease. Ideally, we would image using the highest possible frequency because this would give us the shortest wavelength, enabling excellent axial resolution. However, the increased number of wave fronts results in greater attenuation, and so the sonographer selects a compromise: the highest frequency that is compatible with the required depth of field in the tissue.

The final parameter is the power of sound, measured in decibels (dB). This factor is analogous to the volume of audible sound. It is independent of the velocity, frequency and wavelength.

Production, propagation and detection of ultrasound

Although the terms probe and transducer are often used interchangeably, they are distinct items. The probe is the housing for the transducer, which is the convertor of electronic into vibrational or sound energy, and vice versa. Ultrasound is produced at the surface of the transducer by the piezoelectric effect in thin strips of crystalline material. The elements vibrate for a brief period of time to produce a pulse of sound, which travels into the body. In between the production of sound, the transducer receives the echoes as vibrations, and the reverse piezoelectric effect transforms them into electrical impulses, which make up the monitor display.

Sound is propagated (travels) very well through a perfect homogeneous medium, such as clear water, for example, but, when the wave reaches a material of different density, some of the sound is reflected at the interface. In the body, this happens all the time at the many different interfaces in the tissues, and so there is gradual attenuation of the signal. The sonographer has to optimise the returning signal by the position of the transducer and by use of the instrumentation of the ultrasound machine. These factors mean that sonography is highly dependent on the skill of the operator.

Understanding the ultrasound image

Initially, an image may appear confusing. The first thing to work out is the orientation. This is related to the position of the probe, so only the sonographer knows exactly which plane this is scanning at any one time; this is why it is recommended that the examination be reported by the person who performed it.[1]

The convention for viewing images is that transverse sections are viewed looking towards the head, as in a CT scan, and longitudinal sections are viewed from the subject's right. This is based on a bedside examination where medical staff traditionally stand to the patient's right side and would be the viewpoint of the sonographer in the standard position as shown in **Figure 1.1**, although of course this can be adapted. **Figure 1.2** shows a longitudinal section, seen as if from the patient's right side.

Figure 1.3 also includes a pictogram, a diagram within the image that the sonographer can select to show the exact probe position. Otherwise, an observer can say only that the upper edge of the image is related to the transducer, and beyond this is a slice of increasing depth. Even this may be contradicted when the image is inverted, as may happen in transvaginal sonography or echocardiography.

The differing attenuation patterns are the next area to look at. Fluid-filled areas transmit the sound very well, appearing transonic, or anechoic, meaning there are no echoes returned from within, and resulting in distal acoustic enhancement relative to the adjacent tissues. Conversely, any marked change in density produces a strong reflection,

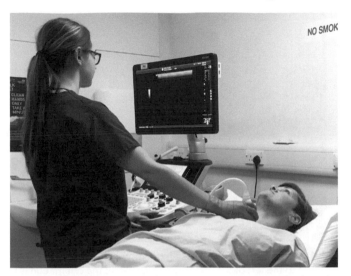

Figure 1.1 The standard ultrasound examination position. Whether the sonographer is left or right handed, both hands are used equally.

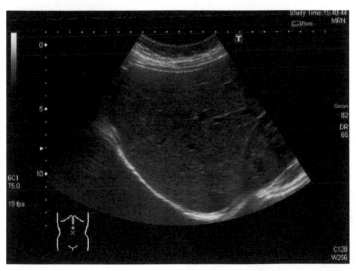

Figure 1.2 A standard longitudinal section of the liver. The diaphragm (superior or cephalad) is to the left of the screen and the kidney (inferior or caudal) is to the right. The anterior surface is at the top of the screen.

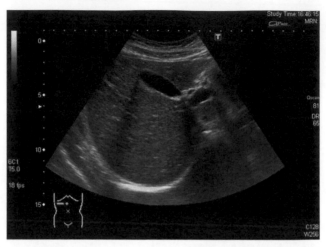

Figure 1.3 A standard transverse section of the liver and gallbladder. The patient's right to the left of the image, and vice versa; the orientation is the same as for viewing computed tomography (CT) and magnetic resonance imaging (MRI) scans.

typically with an acoustic shadow beyond this area (**Figures 1.4 to 1.7**). There is a range of terminology to describe these phenomena: areas that return fewer echoes are often referred to as hypoechoic; those that return no echoes at all may be called anechoic or echo free; and those that send back more echoes and appear brighter are referred to as hyperechoic, and sometimes echogenic.

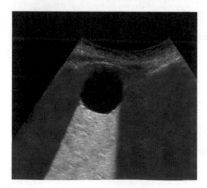

Figure 1.4 Diagrammatic representation of the phenomenon of a fluid area demonstrating posterior acoustic enhancement.

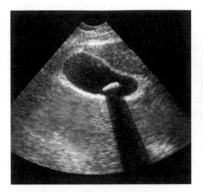

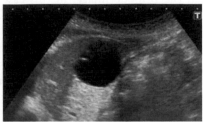

Figure 1.6 A liver cyst, shown as an anechoic or echo-free (black) area with acoustic enhancement (increased brightness) behind it.

Figure 1.5 Diagram of a strong reflector demonstrating acoustic shadowing.

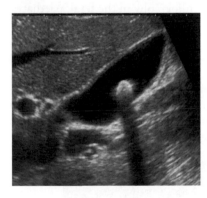

Figure 1.7 A solitary gallstone within the gallbladder. This returns strong (bright) echoes, and so beyond it there is an area of acoustic shadowing, where there is less sound available to generate the image.

Display formats

Even the most basic modern ultrasound machines often come with several display options. The images in **Figures 1.2**, **1.3**, **1.6** and **1.7** are **B mode** images, meaning the signal is brightness modulated, so that the brightness of each pixel is related to the strength of the echo. This gives the familiar greyscale image, which can be seen on all ultrasound monitors.

An **M mode** or movement modulated image displays a single line of the B mode image over time to demonstrate any motion.

The motion of a beating fetal heart is illustrated in **Figure 1.8**, where the tracing shows a spectrum of continuous lines running horizontally along a time base. These lines represent a section along the dotted line in the B mode image; in this case the fetal heart is seen in the near field. The brightness range of the M mode trace corresponds to that in the B mode image, so there are white lines where the beam passes through more reflective tissue and darker areas where it passes through fluid. The depth for each image is shown by the scale at the left of the image; some equipment demonstrates the B mode and the M mode images side by side, which may facilitate viewer orientation. A 'wavy' section of lines can be seen at 3–4 cm depth on the M mode image, and this corresponds to the structure on the B mode image that the dotted line passes through at the same depth (although the image has been 'zoomed' so the superficial 2 cm is not visible). The fetal heart chambers can be seen as fluid areas with the walls appearing brighter, and their movement over time is demonstrated by the M mode trace. M mode is used extensively in echocardiography in the fetal, paediatric and adult fields.

Doppler ultrasound uses the change in frequency when there is relative movement between the sound source and the observer, a phenomenon observed when sound is reflected from a moving object. The signal generated by this frequency shift can be displayed in various ways, depending on the information required. Doppler is often thought to show blood flow, but it should be remembered that it is *movement* that is depicted, as this can give rise to artefactual appearances.

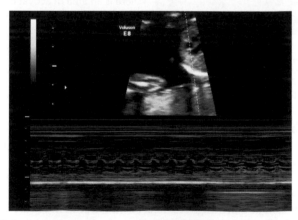

Figure 1.8 An M mode display beneath the corresponding B mode image.

The **spectral Doppler** trace in **Figure** 1.9 shows a series of velocities against a time base. The area sampled is within the Doppler gate, seen as a tiny pair of parallel lines in the corresponding B mode image on the right. The frequency shift of the moving objects within the gate is displayed on the time base to the left, and can also be translated into an audible signal. In this instance, the trace demonstrates the pulsatility of blood flow in the umbilical artery throughout the fetal cardiac cycle.

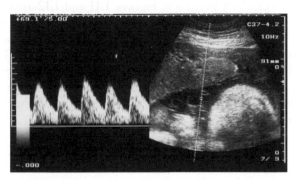

Figure 1.9 A duplex image showing a spectral Doppler trace of an umbilical artery. This is similar to **Figure 1.8** only in that movement is depicted along a time base; the signal processing technology is quite different.

Another type of Doppler display, again obtained by calculation of a shift in frequency between the transmitted pulse and the received echo, is the **colourflow Doppler** image in **Figure** 1.10. Here the shifted frequencies are displayed as a colour 'map' overlay, which is superimposed onto the B mode image. The sample area is in the Doppler box, where all motion is depicted as colour, with the direction and relative speed of flow indicated by a colour scale on the edge of the image. In

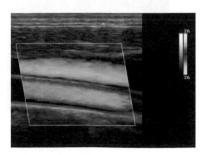

Figure 1.10 A colourflow Doppler image of the neck vessels.

9

this example, the orange colour depicts flow from right to left (carotid artery) and the blue from left to right (jugular vein). The structures must be identified prior to making assumptions about the direction of flow, and this scale must be included in the image in order to interpret the flow and therefore assess anatomy and function.

Power Doppler maps the energy within the image area to give a non-directional display and is excellent for demonstrating low-velocity flow such as capillary perfusion. **Figures 1.11** and **1.12** are comparable images, although from different patients, to illustrate the difference between colourflow and power Doppler. **Figure 1.11** has two distinct colours on the scale, like that in **Figure 1.10**, and shows direction of flow, with an artery and a vein visible within the uterine wall. **Figure 1.12** has a colour continuum and shows the overall vascularity of the myometrium. The applications of Doppler ultrasound are discussed throughout the book and particularly in Chapter 10 on 'The cardio-vascular system'.

Other ultrasound display formats include elastography, where a colour overlay relates to the stiffness of the tissue, useful in tumour recognition and three-dimensional (3D) displays, where the image slices can be digitally reconstructed in the same way that other cross-sectional images permit. There is even four-dimensional (4D) displays where the fourth dimension of time is added to give a real-time 3D image. Elastography is discussed in more detail in Chapter 9 on 'Breast ultrasound'.

All of the above utilise pulsed ultrasound, in which the gaps between the pulses are used to wait for returning echoes. The elapsed time enables the depth registration necessary to produce a display. Although

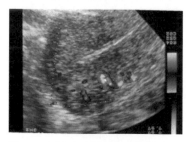

Figure 1.11 A colourflow Doppler image of the uterus.

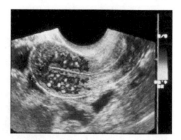

Figure 1.12 A power Doppler image of the uterus.

continuous wave (CW) ultrasound has diagnostic applications, by its nature it is not possible to produce an image from the signal, due to the lack of depth ranging. CW ultrasound is discussed in more detail in the section on ankle–brachial pressure index (ABPI) in Chapter 10 on 'The cardiovascular system'.

Ultrasound equipment, probes and controls

Ultrasound probes are designed with different shapes, sizes and frequency ranges to suit different applications within the body (**Figure 1.13**). Flat-faced linear arrays produce a rectangular image and are useful for superficial structures such as breast and other soft tissues, and for vascular applications. A curved probe face (a curvilinear or convex array) produces a sector-shaped image, so, although near-field visualisation is limited, it combines a good field of view at depth with a smaller 'footprint' for easy access, for instance in abdominal scanning. A phased array (or sector array) has a flat face and a very small footprint but still produces a sector-shaped image; sequential delays are applied to the elements so that it can be set to 'fire' an ultrasound beam in any direction, enabling beam steering in any section, not just along an

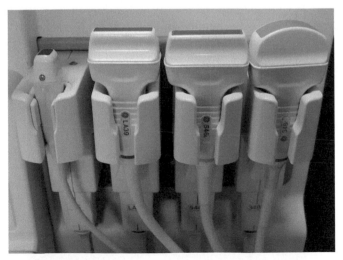

Figure 1.13 A selection of ultrasound probes (left to right): a phased array, two flat linear arrays and a curvilinear probe.

image plane as in linear or curvilinear arrays. Phased arrays are useful in cardiac and neonatal brain scanning. More specialised probes such as endoprobes are discussed in the specific sections where their use is described.

Modern ultrasound transducers are almost all multi-element arrays, which give the option of electronic focusing and beam steering.[2] The elements comprising an array were traditionally tiny strips of quartz, but they are more likely now to be CMUT (capacitive micromachined ultrasonic transducer) or PMUT (piezoelectric micromachined ultrasonic transducer) arrays. They tend to be multi-frequency broadband, so a particular transducer has a range of frequencies, meaning there is no need to change probes when a different frequency is required. It is always best to use the highest possible frequency, as this will give the best possible axial resolution, although the depth of penetration may be reduced. This effect is shown in **Figure 1.14**. On the left, the frequency is 5.5 MHz, giving a smooth image with good resolution; on the right, the frequency of 3 MHz gives much coarser-looking texture to the tissue and poorer resolution. The operator must decrease the frequency for imaging at a greater depth. Lateral resolution is achieved by adjusting the beam focusing to be at the depth of the area of interest (**Figure 1.15**). Good temporal resolution is achieved by optimising the frame rate. This is not generally adjustable itself, but is limited by the depth of view and the number of functions applied by the operator, both of which influence the processing speed of the equipment.

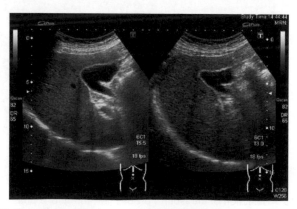

Figure 1.14 The effect of the frequency on resolution in a liver image.

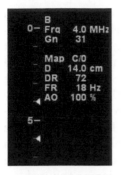

Figure 1.15 A display indicating the equipment settings. The two arrows at 4 and 6 cm depth represent the region of optimum focus, where the beam is narrowest.

The equipment settings and exposure parameters are usually displayed in a corner of the image. Although these vary between manufacturers, **Figure 1.15** shows a typical set of these parameters, and the meaning of these is as follows:

- B – shows the machine is operating with B mode imaging.
- Frq – the transducer is operating at a nominal frequency of 4 MHz, although with a broadband probe this would include slightly higher and lower frequencies too.
- Gn – the overall gain is set at 31 dB.
- Map – this refers to the colour map setting of the display.
- D – depth of field, 14 cm, also displayed on the side scale.
- DR – a dynamic range of 72 dB.
- FR – a frame rate of 18 Hz, as explained above.
- AO – this is the acoustic output, or power setting, which is set at 100% on this image. This may be the manufacturer's default setting, but, in practice, it should be kept as low as possible to minimise any potential bioeffects, while still achieving a diagnostic image. 100% is the maximum and should be used only when absolutely necessary because of these potential bioeffects.

Overall gain, measured in dB, amplifies the echoes uniformly, whereas the time gain compensation (TGC) is applied to preferentially enhance the deeper signals to compensate for the gradual attenuation of the signal through tissue.

TGC is a means of amplification that can be selectively applied to each depth zone because sound from deeper in the body is attenuated more and therefore needs more amplification. The TGC controls are usually a set of slide bars (**Figure 1.16**), where each bar relates to a different depth; the top bars relate to the near field, or more superficial structures, and the lower bars to the far field. The normal default setting is as shown; each slider locates in a central notch, which can be felt as the individual depth control is moved across. Correct adjustment allows visualisation of structures at different depths in an evenly grey image. Although older machines required this to be adjusted manually, manufacturers' presets include an optimum TGC setting for the examination type, which should require only slight adjustment from the centre for most circumstances. The sliders should be reset to the central notches once this extra compensation is no longer required.

The acoustic power increases the transmitted signal and more ultrasound energy enters the patient. When the image is viewed in real time, the amount of transmitted energy is indicated by thermal and mechanical indices, seen as TI and MI, respectively, but these are generally not displayed on the frozen image. The sonographer must understand these figures and keep them as small as possible while setting the controls to optimise the image to a diagnostic quality.[3]

Ultrasound gel is applied to facilitate imaging in three ways: it forms a good acoustic match to ensure that the maximum amount of sound generated is propagated from the transducer to the body part; it

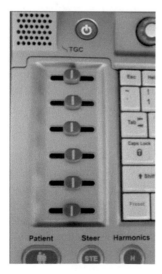

Figure 1.16 Time gain compensation (TGC) controls.

excludes air, again minimising loss of sound; and it enables smoother movement of the probe than may otherwise be possible.

Total quality management (TQM) of a diagnostic ultrasound service

In its broader sense, TQM includes monitoring all aspects of service performance, from response to referrals, through technical aspects of the examination, to reporting delivery and overall patient satisfaction. Thus, TQM incorporates clinical audit and service user feedback as well as technical testing. It is essential to have a departmental scheme of work to set the standards of service and state the protocols for all the different examinations, so that everyone concerned with service provision is aware of their role and responsibilities. Performance guidelines and departmental protocols should be evidence based and compliant with any professional body or national standards, so that there is a clear benchmark of expected performance. Clinical governance is the umbrella term for all of these aspects of performance.

Ultrasound is one of the only imaging modalities where image assessment and diagnosis occur in real time; one of its great strengths is the ability to observe anatomical structures and in some cases functions in real time. Clinical audit programmes need to recognise the subjectivity and operator dependence of ultrasound imaging, and audit should be viewed as a process rather than simply a means to an end, highlighting both areas of good practice and areas where improvement can be made, identifying resources and educational opportunities to maintain standards and enable continual service improvement.[4]

Technical quality assurance (QA) in sonography is a systematic programme to ensure that diagnostic ultrasound instruments are operating consistently at their optimum level of performance. In terms of ultrasound equipment, different levels of quality assurance have been suggested:[5,6]

1. *Acceptance testing on delivery of new equipment* – performed (in the UK National Health Service [NHS]) by the regional medical physics department.
2. *Safety checks prior to each scanning session* – performed by the operator.

3. *Monthly performance tests* – carried out by the ultrasound QA lead or other appropriately trained personnel.
4. *Annual performance checks* – conducted (in the UK NHS) by the regional medical physics department in conjunction with the NHS trust or equipment owner.

Acceptance testing of new equipment, along with annual servicing, are professional services beyond the remit of the sonographer or operator; there are standards laid down for these by the Institute of Physics and Engineering in Medicine.[7]

Thus, the most basic, day-to-day level of QA requires that all equipment users be vigilant for changes that could lead to suboptimal imaging. This requires staff to undertake a visual check of the transducer housing and cables at the start of each session[5] to ensure that the probe is free from cracks in the transducer housing or damage to the membranous face covering.

Surface damage to the rubberised membrane that covers the transducer face is shown in **Figure 1.17**. In the corresponding sonogram (**Figure 1.18**) the linear dark artefact is due to crystal damage at this point, resulting in a loss of part of the image.

Probe damage may result from physical abuse such as dropping the probe or repeatedly replacing it face down in its holster or, worst of

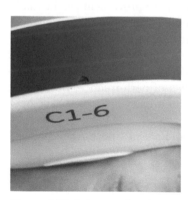

Figure 1.17 A damaged probe surface.

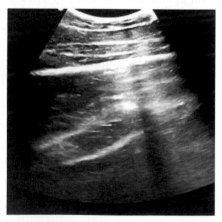

Figure 1.18 A sonogram produced with the same probe.

all, leaving it draped and hanging, which should never occur. A lack of probe housing integrity can be an infection as well as an electrical risk.

The operator should also be vigilant for any changes in image quality, such as loss of scan lines due to individual crystal damage, as seen in **Figure 1.19**. This probe has several areas of crystal damage with loss of the scan lines from these points; this is colloquially known as 'crystal drop out'. The probe that produced this image was condemned by the medical physics department on inspection. Another visible change in image quality is 'ghosting' of the on-screen text, suggesting a lack of sharpness within the image.

Transducer cables comprise very many, sometimes hundreds, of tiny wires, and are highly vulnerable to damage when run over by the cart itself during manoeuvring into position. This must never happen! The best way of ensuring equipment longevity is for the operator to ensure that the probes and cables are correctly stowed at the end of each examination to protect them from damage.

The monthly performance tests are more objective than the daily visual checks and are carried out using a test object or tissue equivalent 'phantom'. This is essentially a scannable box containing various items such as wires at a known distance apart or structures of a specific known size and depth, as shown in **Figures 1.20** and **1.21**. The calliper (measurement) accuracy and the axial and lateral resolution of the beam can be checked by on-screen measurements of a sonogram of this object, producing an image such as that in **Figure 1.22**. The results should be logged so that any change over time can be identified, often before an obvious equipment malfunction occurs.

Additional QA measures may be applicable in certain circumstances, for instance in screening programmes, or in vascular services where

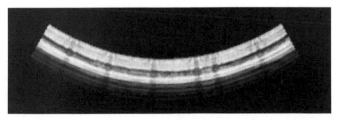

Figure 1.19 Loss of several scan lines, visible in the near-field reverberations even when not scanning an object.

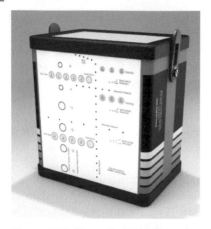

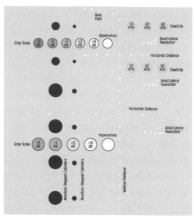

Figure 1.20 This is the CIRS (Computerized Imaging Reference Systems, Inc.) tissue equivalent test object, model 040GSE, known as a 'phantom'.

Figure 1.21 Manufacturer's diagram of the interior of CIRS 040GSE.

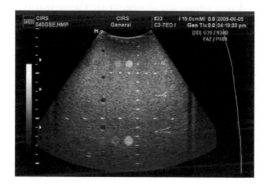

Figure 1.22 A sonogram of the CIRS 040GSE.

specialised checks for Doppler ultrasound may be made, and for monitors where images are to be viewed remotely.[8] As in other branches of imaging, only medical-grade monitors should be used for image interpretation and these should be subject to a QA programme to check for any drifting from their optimal settings or performance. Such processes and systems ensure that image quality is optimal and data measurements are accurate, helping to provide confidence in the service provided.

Advantages of ultrasound as a modality

- The equipment is relatively inexpensive and so is readily available.
- The equipment is generally mobile and may be portable.
- Examination times are short and with little necessity for preparation.
- Ultrasound scanning is a non-invasive modality that does not involve ionising radiation.
- Immediate, accurate measurements (biometry) are available.
- Real-time visualisation enables evaluation of movement, compressibility of tissue, and guidance of instruments in surgery or other interventions (see Chapter 12 'The central nervous system – eye and brain').
- This ability to visualise movement means that subject motion does not unduly detract from the image quality.
- High manoeuvrability and unlimited angulation allow access in difficult circumstances, for example in trauma, during surgical operations or when dressings or other artefactual objects limit access.
- Vascular imaging including biometry is possible with spectral, colourflow and power Doppler to evaluate vascular supply, drainage and anomalies.

Disadvantages of ultrasound as a modality

- Ultrasound is a highly operator-dependent modality, relying heavily on the skill of the sonographer to interpret the clinical history in order to image the correct structures, using the best equipment settings, and observing and recording the relevant findings. Therefore, a high standard of sonographic education is required to practise. Continuing clinical audit and assistance from artificial intelligence (AI) may help to ensure quality of examinations.
- Because it is very much a 'real-time' modality, interpretation is best made during the procedure itself. A retrospective review of the images or even a real-time recording cannot capture the whole examination, and the potential for evaluation of movement or compressibility is lost in a recording.
- Ultrasound does not travel through gas – for example in bowel, through clothes or dressings or in abscesses.
- Limitations are possible with larger or more solid subjects due to sound attenuation.

Comparison with other imaging modalities

- As compared with CT scanning, ultrasound gives better temporal resolution and good contrast resolution when the equipment settings are optimised, but has poorer spatial resolution.
- The contrast resolution is better in MRI, but the good temporal resolution of ultrasound, along with the ease of access and possible use of metal equipment, makes ultrasound-guided interventions much more practical.
- Generally, nuclear medicine is better than ultrasound for organ function, although ultrasound yields better detail in real time of many of the body's functions, for example peristalsis, blood flow or in obstetric imaging.

Overall, ultrasound equipment is cheaper and more portable than CT, MRI or nuclear medicine equipment, and is widely used in every sphere of medicine from battlegrounds to high-altitude emergency care, for diagnostic imaging and sampling as well as surgical guidance, line placements, drainages and therapeutic drug delivery. Developments in fusion imaging show promise for future tissue characterisation, as discussed in Chapter 15 'Additional technologies'.

Ultrasound in screening programmes

Due to its advantages, ultrasound is the imaging modality employed in the UK for the Fetal Anomaly Screening Programme (NHS FASP) and the National Abdominal Aortic Aneurysm Screening Programme (NAAASP). In the NHS Breast Screening Programme (NHS BSP), it is more useful as a follow-up examination at present. Ultrasound is also widely used in targeted screening of individuals in affected families for polycystic kidney disease and ovarian cancer screening, and for neonates with possible hip dysplasia as part of the Newborn and Infant Physical Examination (NIPE) screening programme.

PATIENT PREPARATION AND CARE

Preparation for the examination

For many ultrasound examinations, no special physical preparation is needed. One exception is imaging of the upper abdominal organs, where bowel gas is an impediment to good sonographic imaging because the high-frequency and therefore short-wavelength ultrasound cannot travel through gas, including air. Bowel gas is a normal result of chewing and swallowing, so restriction of eating and drinking is commonly used to try to reduce it. This is known as 'fasting' or 'starving'.

Even more important is the requirement for the biliary system to be in its relaxed state for optimum visualisation and accurate measurement of the common duct during investigation of the liver and biliary system. To achieve this state, patients are often asked to abstain from food and drink for around 4–6 hours prior to their examination.[9] In fact, a regime of fat-free food and drink may be sufficient, but it is often simpler to ask for complete fasting. Longer periods of fasting are unwarranted and may be detrimental to patient health.[10]

The other useful patient preparation is filling of the urinary bladder for transabdominal pelvic examinations. A full urinary bladder helps in imaging the pelvic organs by acting as an acoustic window and a landmark, while displacing bowel and therefore gas, and by moving the uterus in the female pelvis into a more accessible position. A full bladder may be achieved by the patient taking ~900 ml (a pint and a half) of still water or other still liquid an hour before the examination; this allows time for the fluid to reach the bladder. A bladder volume of 350–500 ml is usually sufficient to perform the investigation. If the patient is scanned too soon after drinking, the fluid may be in the small bowel and prevent clear visualisation. Fizzy drinks can produce an excess of bowel gas with a similar effect. Under-filling may yield suboptimal images, whereas over-filling or waiting too long may cause considerable discomfort, as well as a false appearance of hydronephrosis if the kidneys are to be examined at the same time.

Unlike most other imaging modalities, an ultrasound examination is not possible through any clothing, which therefore needs to be removed and a gown offered as a covering garment where required.

The sonographer should be able to access the body for the examination while ensuring privacy is maintained with skilful manipulation of gowns, blankets, paper towels and other coverings. It is possible to preserve dignity at all times with appropriate care. Jewellery should be removed if it is likely to become covered in gel or cause an obstruction to visualisation. Wound dressings or bandages must also be removed for direct access and, if this is not possible, their presence may be a contraindication to sonographic examination.

It is common to warm the coupling gel to lessen the shock of its application, although this may contribute to an environment where microbial growth is possible.[11] Single-use pre-filled gel bottles should be used, and sterile single-use sachets of gel should be available for sterile procedures. The use of gel, the necessary operator–patient skin contact and the possibility of infections and/or open wounds mean that the utmost attention must be paid to infection control measures in any ultrasound examination.[12]

Communication in sonography

Good communication skills are essential in sonography. The procedure should always be fully explained before starting, not only as a courtesy to the patient, but also because cooperation is required to execute a high-quality examination. Sonography differs from most other imaging modalities apart from fluoroscopy in that the subject and the operator are in close proximity and can often see each other's faces as the image is produced. The patient may well try to deduce what is happening, sometimes wrongly, if the operator does not explain the procedure or at least say that the examination may take some time and require the utmost concentration, which may preclude conversation. Communication is therefore key to a quality sonogram and of course a prerequisite for informed consent.[13]

Valid consent is part of person-centred care and should be obtained for any examination. The patient should be provided with information about the procedure prior to the examination. When they arrive in the scan room, it is important that the sonographer ensures that the patient understands the voluntary nature of the procedure in addition to:

- details of the examination;
- the benefits and limitations of the examination;
- any consequences of not having the test;
- possible alternative options available;
- any potential side effects or risks.

For example, when explaining a transvaginal scan, it is important to ensure that: the patient is fully aware that the scan can give better visualisation of the uterus, endometrium and ovaries, but is optional; the decontaminated probe will be covered with a probe cover and will have a small amount of gel on the end to help smooth insertion; the probe will be inserted into the vagina, and they can insert it themselves or the sonographer can do that. Once in the vagina, the probe will be moved slightly from side to side and up and down, which might be uncomfortable but should not be painful. If there is any pain or if the patient has any questions or wants the procedure to be stopped, they just need to say so. Providing clear communication before, during and after the procedure will reduce the chance of misunderstanding and complaints.

Valid consent presumes that the adult has capacity to consent, in so much as they can:

- understand the information provided;
- retain that information long enough to decide;
- review the benefits and risks of having the procedure;
- clearly communicate their decision to the practitioner.

The UK Department of Health and Social Care (DHSC) advises that 'consent is usually a process, rather than a one-off event'. It is essential to check that consent is continuing for a procedure as you progress through an examination. There are specific guidelines for children and those with limited capacity to consent, with which sonographers should be familiar.[14,15]

Delivering unexpected findings

One of the most difficult parts of a sonographer's role can be communicating the ultrasound findings to patients. There are many occasions, not just in obstetrics, when unexpected findings must be communicated to the patient. Sonographers should be aware of the approaches

Avoid assumptions	• We are unaware of what the findings will mean for individual patients. • Talk in neutral terms, rather than saying 'I am sorry', as this assumes that it's bad news.
Set up the scan	• Before the examination, try to find out what the patient expectations are and clarify any additional points. • Explain during the consent process any issues that could potentially arise, e.g. the need for an alternative technique, investigation, rescan or blood test. • Discuss how the results will be delivered.
Clear, honest information	• Information should be clear and honest. Avoid the use of jargon. • Provide information in small chunks, then wait and check understanding before giving any further information. • Use eye contact. • In some cases, it may be appropriate to discuss the findings on the screen, but remember to give the patient a choice. • Explain what will happen next. • If you are not the appropriate person to give further information, say so but also signpost the patient to that person. • Provide written information where possible.
Kindness	• Show empathy and compassion. • Use the terms that the patient uses. • Give patients time to process the information. • If appropriate, express regret. Remember this might not always be appropriate, so wait until you find out how the information is received.
Self care	• Self-care, support and developing your own coping mechanisms are all important tools for sonographers.

Figure 1.23 ASCKS framework for delivering unexpected news in obstetric ultrasound.[16]

that might be used to ensure that the patient fully understands the information and what the next steps are. The chart (**Figure 1.23**) shows an adaptation of the ASCKS approach to delivering unexpected findings or difficult news in obstetric ultrasound.[16]

Sometimes the consent process can aid in preparing patients for unequivocal findings, for example the early pregnancy patient that needs to come back for a rescan in 2 weeks, when the gestation sac is too small to determine whether there is a developing pregnancy. Before starting the scan, as part of informed consent, the sonographer could say: *'Sometimes in the early stages of pregnancy it may be difficult to see the pregnancy sac or baby. If this is the case, we may need to check again in 2 weeks' time.'* When discussing the findings, a 'warning shot' that something unusual is about to be explained could be, for instance: *'At the beginning of the scan I said that sometimes we need to arrange another scan if the sac is too small to see a baby; well that is the case with your pregnancy today'*. This works equally well in other situations where alternative imaging may be required, for example the scenario where a patient is attending for an abdominal scan to look for secondary spread. The sonographer could, during the consent process, say that: *'Ultrasound is often the first test that we do, sometimes other examinations may be needed.'*

As a general rule, it is preferable to discuss findings with patients at the same height as the sonographer and to maintain eye contact. If an interpreter is used, they should ideally sit slightly behind the sonographer's shoulder. That way both the sonographer and the interpreter can maintain eye contact with the patient at all times during the conversation. In some situations, it can be helpful for patients to see the findings on the monitor as they are being discussed. It is important to ask the patient for their views before deciding which is the most appropriate method, for example: *'I would like to discuss the findings of the scan with you. Would you prefer to get dressed and sit up or would you like me to show you on the screen?'*

When explaining findings to patients and their relatives, it is essential to provide clear, honest explanations, while working within the individual sonographer's scope of practice and level of competency. If a sonographer does not know the answer to a question, it is far better to say so and signpost the patient to someone who might be able to answer the question than to give incorrect or confusing information. During the discussions, continuously check whether the explanations are clear and provide small amounts of information at a time. Often patients go into shock and may need time to process the news. It can be helpful to remain silent, to give patients time to assimilate the information being provided. Rather than ask a patient if they understand what you are saying, it is better to say something such as: '*Am I explaining this clearly enough for you?*' That way they do not feel at fault if they are finding it difficult to take in the information.

Self-care and good peer support are essential for sonographers. Talking to colleagues and general debriefs can be useful.

SAFETY CONSIDERATIONS

Scheme of work – protocols

Each facility should have a scheme of work, stating the sonographers' roles and responsibilities and outlining the scope of practice. This may include writing the clinical report, providing an interpretation of the findings, correlating the clinical details provided, recommending further investigations including X-ray, CT, MRI and blood tests, and communicating the findings verbally to clinicians, patients and carers. Additionally, protocols should provide detailed information about the areas to be scanned and reported for each body part or examination type. Protocols should be evidence based, dated clearly and updated regularly. As new protocols are introduced, the old protocols should be archived, as they may need to be referred to in the future.

Safety considerations

Bioeffects of ultrasound have been demonstrated in vitro, and the principle of ALARP ('as low as reasonably practicable') should be used, as in any imaging procedure. The use of Doppler ultrasound is not advised within the developing embryo, as this is potentially the highest intensity mode and the most vulnerable scenario. M mode is a lower energy alternative that is much under-used and should be considered as a better means of demonstrating cardiac activity.[17] Otherwise, no detrimental effects of normal intensity diagnostic ultrasound have been proven in clinical use.

However, sonography is not without its risks, and these include:

■ *Psychological considerations* – sonography by its intimate nature may lead to communication issues, as outlined in this chapter in the section 'Patient preparation and care'.

■ *Operator error* – the greatest danger to the patient is misdiagnosis because the results of a sonogram rely solely on the operator(s) in terms of image acquisition, optimisation, recording and interpretation. Anyone who carries out an ultrasound examination must be aware not only of their skills but also of their limitations, and not proceed beyond these.

■ *Infection* – because of the necessity for bare skin contact, the use of scanning gel, which may become a contaminant, and the proximity of operator and subject, cross-infection, whether between patients or between the operator and the patient, is a real risk, and very high standards of infection control are therefore required.[11] All types of endocavity sonograms in particular should have a specific protocol for infection prevention and control procedures to reduce or eliminate infection exposure to the patient, operator and equipment.[18] Sterile gel rather than standard clean gel must be used:
  – for invasive procedures, such as amniocentesis or biopsy;
  – where there is contact with wounds or other broken skin;
  – during endocavity procedures;
  – for examinations on neonates and immunocompromised or critically ill patients in intensive care or other high-dependency settings.

■ When an operator wears latex medical gloves or when probe covers are used, as in endocavity examinations, it is important to check if the patient has a latex allergy. Vinyl alternatives should be available in case of allergy or for the unconscious patient.

■ Sonographers themselves are at high risk of work-related musculoskeletal disorders, due to the physical and repetitive nature of the examination.[19] All training should include advice on how to optimise the ergonomics and minimise risk of strain.[20]

Decontamination of ultrasound equipment

It is important, after every examination, to decontaminate the ultrasound machine and probes carefully to reduce the chance of cross-contamination between patients. Two alerts relating to ultrasound probes have been published, highlighting the risks to patients of inappropriate decontamination.[21,22] Decontamination levels will depend on the nature of the examination and contact with patient body parts, for example intact skin, broken or infected skin surfaces, endocavity examinations or intraoperative procedures. For any procedure, immediately after the examination is completed the probe should be wiped clean of any visible matter (**Figure 1.24**). If gel or other material is not removed before disinfection or sterilisation of the probe, the procedure can be less effective.

Manufacturer-approved products must be used when selecting which is the most appropriate method of decontaminating each individual probe to prevent damage. Local infection control teams should also be involved in discussion about the optimal methods for every examination type. In some cases, different products are needed for the probe compared with the machine and cables. Automated systems are recommended as best practice for disinfection of endocavity probes or probes that have been in contact with broken or infected skin or patients with known infections.[23]

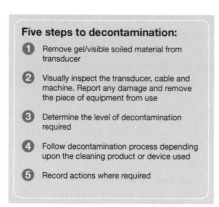

Five steps to decontamination:

1. Remove gel/visible soiled material from transducer

2. Visually inspect the transducer, cable and machine. Report any damage and remove the piece of equipment from use

3. Determine the level of decontamination required

4. Follow decontamination process depending upon the cleaning product or device used

5. Record actions where required

Figure 1.24 Transducer decontamination: best practice summary.[18]

For any decontamination process it is important that all staff are fully trained, audited and comply with local protocols. For disinfection and sterilisation the process should be documented clearly for each patient interaction, to ensure that a full audit trail is available should there be any future issues.[18]

Work-related musculoskeletal disorders (WRMSDs)

WRMSDs are prevalent among sonographers, so it is important to consider ways to reduce the chance of injury. There are many factors that can help protect sonographers and a plethora of research and guidance is available (see the literature [19,24,25]).

Employers have a responsibility to ensure that the workplace is safe and provide appropriate equipment to protect sonographers. This includes ergonomic equipment such as a movable couch and appropriate chair that supports the sonographer to sit upright and get as close to the patient as possible. Other factors that impact on WRMSDs are workload pressures, patient obesity or mobility, psychosocial factors and stress, poor management and lack of control over workload.[20]

Key considerations when planning the ultrasound workload are:

- Room design to ensure enough space to optimise the scanning position.
- Mixed ultrasound examination lists where possible, to vary the workload and posture.
- Provision of breaks allow sonographers to refocus their eyes, stretch and relax. Microbreaks such as resting the scanning hand for a few seconds while taking a measurement can be helpful to allow muscle recovery.
- Risk assessments should be undertaken for each sonographer and examination type, as risks will vary for individual circumstances.

Ergonomics includes the ability of the sonographer to adapt the equipment and tasks to suit them and their needs, rather than working around the equipment. Good ergonomic education and understanding are central to reducing the chance of WRMSDs.

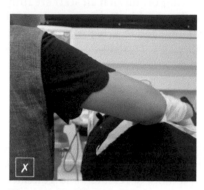

Figure 1.25 The arm is abducted (>30°); this puts strain on the shoulder.

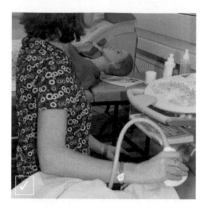

Figure 1.26 The shoulder is vertical, the upper arm is close to the body (<30°) and the forearm is horizontal.

There are many things that sonographers can do to reduce injury, such as:

- Set the top of the monitor to allow free movement of the neck. Slightly flexed or neutral position of the neck, rather than extended, is optimal.
- Keep the scanning arm close to the body, reducing arm abduction to less than 30° (Figures 1.25 and 1.26).
- Ensure the forearm of the scanning arm is horizontal (Figure 1.26).
- Use a power grip or modified power grip (Figure 1.26), rather than a pinch grip (Figure 1.27), when holding the transducer.
- Reduce wrist flexion and extension and hand deviation to a minimum. Moving the whole arm or forearm sometimes helps to reduce hand and wrist movements.

Move the chair backwards if the arm is extended slightly behind the body (Figure 1.28). The optimal position of the shoulder is such that the upper arm is vertical and close to the side of the body (Figure 1.26). Note that jewellery should not be worn when scanning, to reduce cross-infection.

Sonographers can improve their general well-being and reduce the risks to themselves by warming up before a scanning session, for instance with body twists and arm swings, stretching between patients

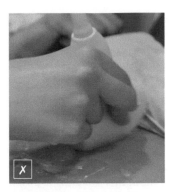

Figure 1.27 Pinch grip: this strains the fingers. All four fingers should be used to hold the probe and the grip should be relaxed, so there are no white knuckles.

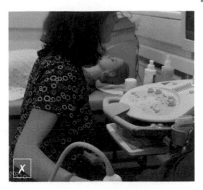

Figure 1.28 The shoulder demonstrates posterior extension, putting additional strain on the shoulder. If the chair is moved back slightly this would optimise the position.

and at the end of the ultrasound list, and building upper body strength and keeping fit.[26]

Clinical report writing

Report writing is an integral part of the examination and should not be separated from the ultrasound scan, because the operator builds up a 3D image in their mind as they undertake the scan, and this cannot be captured by still images or even video. In the UK, professional guidelines state that the operator should interpret and report the findings of an ultrasound examination.[1,27]

The report should communicate the findings of the examination in a clear and concise way to reduce errors in interpretation and the medicolegal consequences of misinterpretation. Sonographers should be aware of best practice guidance from the Society and College of Radiographers (SCoR), the British Medical Ultrasound Society (BMUS) and The Royal College of Radiologists (RCR). If a structure appears normal, the sonographer should report this. It is recommended that the present tense be used throughout the report and consistency of units of measurement used, for example: '*The uterus appears normal, measuring 73 mm × 40 mm × 31 mm. The endometrial cavity appears normal with an endometrial thickness of 6 mm.*'

When writing, tautology (repetition of words) should be avoided, for example: *'both ovaries seen and appear normal'* – if they appear normal, they have been seen; *'abnormally dilated'* – if a structure is dilated it is abnormal. Also, the report should not include 'hedging' statements such as: *'no obvious'*. If it were obvious, the sonographer would have seen and reported it. It would be preferable to conclude: *'normal examination'* or *'normal ultrasound appearances'*.

Clinicians reading the report may not understand ultrasound terminology so the sonographer should make sure to provide clear information, avoiding the use of jargon and providing an interpretation of any description, for example: *'the gallbladder contains a 23 mm mobile, shadowing hyperechoic focus'* would be better described as: *'the gallbladder contains a mobile gallstone, measuring 23 mm'*.

The report should include the information as shown in the text boxes at the end of this section, in addition to patient details.

Sonographers must work within their scope of practice. If unsure of how to word a report or interpret the findings, a second opinion should be sought from a colleague. This should be included within the report, for example *'Findings discussed with Dr X, who recommends follow-up CT scan'*. Any further actions by the sonographer should be documented, for example discussing the findings with the general practitioner (GP) or referring the patient to the early pregnancy assessment unit. Communication of findings with the patient may also be recorded within the report.

There are a number of standardised reporting tools available for different clinical areas, to develop consistency of report writing. These include the American College of Radiology (ACR) Reporting and Data Systems (RADS) and the International Ovarian Tumor Analysis (IOTA) definitions.[28]

Clinical details and examination procedure:

- Brief summary of the clinical details, including the clinical question to be answered
- Any other relevant information gained from the patient, for example last menstrual period, additional relevant symptoms
- Type of examination (e.g. transabdominal, transvaginal or transrectal)
- Persons present, for example other staff, students, relatives, chaperone; include whether a chaperone was offered and accepted or declined
- Known allergies (if latex products are used in the department/clinic) and precautions

Examination findings:

- Normal appearances, for example: *'the liver, spleen and pancreas appear normal'*
- When quoting measurements state whether they are normal or not. If the report is for a general practitioner, it is also helpful to state the normal expected measurement to give some context, for example: *'the common duct appears dilated, measuring 9 mm (normal max. 6 mm)'*
- Shape, size, outline and echotexture of abnormalities, along with other findings such as vascularity, mass effect, spread or attenuation, for example: *'the liver is homogeneously bright in echotexture and highly attenuating, suggestive of fatty change'*
- Mention any limitations of the examination, but only if they impact on the diagnosis. This helps the clinician decide if other investigations are needed, for example: *'the head and body of pancreas appear normal, the tail is obscured by bowel gas'*

Conclusion:

- Provide a conclusion, which interprets the findings. Answer the clinical question, but do not repeat the detail, for example: *'Conclusion: Appearances are consistent with gallstones'*
- Where possible give a diagnosis or differential diagnoses and suggestions for further examinations, for example: *'Conclusion: Appearances are suggestive of an FNH or adenoma. CEUS or MRI would be advised to differentiate'*
- State any management or referral suggestions, if applicable and relevant, depending on the referrer, for example: *'Suggest urgent urology referral'*

Examiner details:

- Ensure that the name and role/designation of the operator and/or reporter and any other relevant information is provided on the report
- The Royal College of Radiologists (RCR) recommends that the registration number be provided for a registered healthcare professional within the report

REFERENCES

1. SCoR (Society and College of Radiographers), BMUS (British Medical Ultrasound Society). *Guidelines for professional ultrasound practice.* London: SCoR and BMUS, 2021. Available at: https://www.sor.org/learning-advice/professional-body-guidance-and-publications/documents-and-publications/policy-guidance-document-library.
2. Szabo TL, Lewin PA. Ultrasound transducer selection in clinical imaging practice. *Journal of Ultrasound in Medicine* 2013;**32**(4):573–582. doi: 10.7863/jum.2013.32.4.573.

3. RCR (Royal College of Radiologists), SCoR (Society and College of Radiographers). *Standards for the provision of an ultrasound service.* London: RCR, 2014. Available at: https://www.rcr.ac.uk/system/files/publication/field_publication_files/BFCR(14)17_Standards_ultrasound.pdf.

4. ter Haar G (ed.). *The safe use of ultrasound in medical diagnosis,* 3rd edn. London: The British Institute of Radiology, 2012. Available at: http://www.birpublications.org/pb/assets/raw/Books/SUoU_3rdEd/Safe_Use_of_Ultrasound.pdf.

5. Dudley N, Russell S, Ward B, Hoskins P; BMUS QA Working Party. BMUS guidelines for the regular quality assurance testing of ultrasound scanners by sonographers. *Ultrasound* 2014 Feb;**22**(1):8–14. doi: 10.1177/1742271X13511805.

6. Dudley N, Woolley D. Diagnostic ultrasound quality assurance manual. 2021. Multi-Medix. Available via https://multi-medix.com/us/quality-assurance/

7. IPEM (The Institute of Physics and Engineering in Medicine). *Report 102 quality assurance of ultrasound imaging systems.* York: IPEM, 2010.

8. Kagadis GC, Walz-Flannigan A, Krupinski EA, Nagy PG, Katsanos K, Diamantopoulos A, Langer SG. Medical image displays and their use in image interpretation. *Radiographics* 2013;**33**(1):275–290. doi: 10.1148/rg.331125096.

9. Ehrenstein BP, Froh S, Schlottmann K, Schölmerich J, Schacherer D. To eat or not to eat? Effect of fasting prior to abdominal sonography examinations on the quality of imaging under routine conditions: A randomized, examiner-blinded trial. *Scandinavian Journal of Gastroenterology.* 2009;**44**(9):1048–1054. doi: 10.1080/00365520903075188.

10. Lamb S, Close A, Bonnin C, Ferrie S. 'Nil by mouth' – Are we starving our patients? *e-SPEN the European e-Journal of Clinical Nutrition and Metabolism* 2010;**5**(2):e90–e92. doi: 10.1016/j.eclnm.2010.01.003.

11. Muradali D, Gold WL, Phillips A, Wilson S. Can ultrasound probes and coupling gel be a source of nosocomial infection in patients undergoing sonography? An in vivo and in vitro study. *American Journal of Roentgenology* 1995;**164**(6):1521–1524. doi: 10.2214/AJR.164.6.7754907.

12. Tunstall TD. Infection control in the sonography department. *Journal of Diagnostic Medical Sonography* 2010;**26**(4):190–197. doi: 10.1177/8756479310374362.

13. HCPC (Health and Care Professions Council). Standards of conduct, performance and ethics. Health and Care Professions Council, 2016. Available at: https://www.hcpc-uk.org/globalassets/resources/standards/standards-of-conduct-performance-and-ethics.pdf

14. DHSC (Department of Health & Social Care). *Reference guide to consent for examination or treatment*, 2nd edn. London: DHSC, 2009. Available at: https://assets.publishing.service.gov.uk/government/uploads/system/uploads/attachment_data/file/138296/dh_103653__1_.pdf.

15. SCoR (Society and College of Radiographers). *Obtaining consent: A clinical guideline for the diagnostic imaging and radiotherapy workforce*. London: SCoR, 2020. Available at: https://www.sor.org/getmedia/d0f41e69-2006-43a8-9c75-1dae2ad04c69/work_related_musculoskeletal_disorders_sonographers-pdf_3

16. Johnson J, Arezina J, Tomlin L, Alt S, Arnold J, Bailey S, et al. UK consensus guidelines for the delivery of unexpected news in obstetric ultrasound: The ASCKS framework. *Ultrasound* 2020;**28**(4):235–245. doi: 10.1177/1742271X20935911.

17. RCOG (Royal College of Obstetricians and Gynaecologists). *Ultrasound from conception to 10 + 0 weeks of gestation (Scientific Impact Paper No. 49)*. London: RCOG, 2015. Available at: https://www.rcog.org.uk/globalassets/documents/guidelines/scientific-impact-papers/sip-49.pdf.

18. AXREM, BMUS, SCoR. *Ultrasound transducer decontamination – best practice summary*. AXREM, 2020. Available at: https://www.axrem.org.uk/resource/ultrasound-transducer-decontamination-best-practice-summary/.

19. Dodgeon J, Newton-Hughes A. Are you sitting comfortably? Enabling sonographers to minimise work-related musculoskeletal disorders. *British Medical Ultrasound Society Bulletin* 2003;**11**(3):16–21. doi: 10.1177/1742271X0301100304.

20. Harrison G, Harris A. Work-related musculoskeletal disorders in ultrasound: Can you reduce risk? *Ultrasound* 2015;**23**(4):224–230. doi: 10.1177/1742271X15593575.

21. MHPRA (Medicines and Healthcare Products Regulatory Agency). *Ultrasound transducer probes with an internal lumen used for taking transrectal prostate biopsies*. London: MHPRA, 2009. Available at: https://assets.publishing.service.gov.uk/media/5485ac42ed915d4c100002a7/con065543.pdf.

22. MHPRA (Medicines and Healthcare Products Regulatory Agency). *Reusable transoesophageal echocardiography, transvaginal and transrectal ultrasound probes (transducers) – failure to appropriately decontaminate*. London: MHPRA, 2014. Available at: https://www.gov.uk/drug-device-alerts/medical-device-alert-reusable-transoesophageal-echocardiography-transvaginal-and-transrectal-ultrasound-probes-transducers-failure-to-appropriately-decontaminate.

23. Bradley C, Hoffman P, Egan K, Jacobson S. Guidance for the decontamination of intracavity medical devices: The report of a working group of the Healthcare Infection Society. *Journal of Hospital Infection* 2018;**101**(3):1–10. doi: 10.1016/j.jhin.2018.08.003.

24. Monnington S, Dodd-Hughes K, Milnes E, Ahmad Y. *Project report: Risk management of musculoskeletal disorders in sonography work.* Cardiff: Health and Safety Executive, 2012. http://www.hse.gov.uk/healthservices/management-of-musculoskeletal-disorders-in-sonography-work.pdf.

25. SCoR (Society and College of Radiographers). *Work related musculoskeletal disorders (sonographers)*, 3rd edn. London: SCoR, 2019. Available at: https://www.sor.org/getmedia/d0f41e69-2006-43a8-9c75-1dae2ad04c69/work_related_musculoskeletal_disorders_sonographers-pdf_3.

26. Leah C. *Exercises to reduce musculoskeletal discomfort for people doing a range of static and repetitive work.* London: HSE, 2011. https://www.hse.gov.uk/research/rrpdf/rr743.pdf.

27. CASE. *Standards for sonographic education 2019: Consortium for the Accreditation of Sonographic Education.* 2019. Available at: http://www.case-uk.org/standards/.

28. Timmerman D, Valentin L, Bourne TH, Collins WP. International Ovarian Tumor Analysis (IOTA) Group. Terms, definitions and measurements to describe the sonographic features of adnexal tumors: A consensus opinion from the International Ovarian Tumor Analysis (IOTA) Group. *Ultrasound in Obstetrics and Gynecology* 2000;**16**(5):500–505. doi: 10.1046/j.1469-0705.2000.00287.x.

Further reading

Dudley N. *Diagnostic ultrasound quality assurance manual.* Multi-Medix, 2020. Available at: https://multi-medix.com/diagnostic-ultrasound-quality-assurance-manual/.

Gibbs V, Cole D, Sassano A. *Ultrasound physics and technology: How, why and when.* Edinburgh: Churchill-Livingstone, 2009.

Sanders R, Winter T. *Clinical sonography.* 4th edn. London: Lippincott Williams & Wilkins, 2006.

CHAPTER 2

THE UPPER ABDOMINAL ORGANS

The pancreas   43
The liver and biliary system   48
The portal venous system   55
The spleen   58
References   63

Patient preparation and care

Ultrasound is the first-line investigation for a range of upper abdominal complaints due to its non-invasive nature, meaning it has high patient acceptability as well as being readily available. It is an excellent tool for imaging the liver, gallbladder and spleen, and is used for the diagnosis and monitoring of various conditions. Ultrasound is relatively cost-effective when compared with other imaging modalities such as computed tomography (CT) and magnetic resonance imaging (MRI).

The patient should fast for 4–6 hours prior to the examination to ensure that the gallbladder is in a relaxed (non-contracted) state and to try to avoid any gut content that might obscure the areas of interest.[1] The portal vein diameter varies depending on the time after the last meal.[2] Only a small amount of water or other clear fluid is advised to retain hydration without filling the stomach.

Talking to the patient will enable acquisition of a detailed history while helping to put the patient at ease. As always, valid, informed consent to the examination should be gained, and this includes the need to explain the limitations of ultrasound, particularly for the assessment of the pancreas. It is common for patients with pancreatic pathology to require further imaging such as CT. Explanation prior to the examination can reduce patient anxiety if further examinations are required. Information is important when using spectral Doppler because the noise made when assessing the vessel may alarm the patient. Clothing should be removed from the area under examination. Privacy and dignity should be maintained throughout the examination. Paper towels can be used to protect the patient's clothing from the coupling gel applied to the region being examined.

Upper abdominal organs should always be scanned together, not in isolation, because they are functionally connected. A disease process in one organ may result in complications in the other organs and symptoms, such as epigastric pain, may arise from pathology in any of these organs. It is recommended that an upper abdominal examination be started with the pancreas for two reasons. First, the pancreas may become obscured by gas as the patient lies supine for some time, so early access is more likely to provide clear visualisation and second, as the pancreas can be difficult to image, it will be possible to return to it at the end of the examination, if necessary.

Liver and biliary system: blood tests

Jaundice can be caused by many different pathologies. The main role of ultrasound in assessing a patient with jaundice is to determine whether there is an obstructive or non-obstructive cause. Causes of non-obstructive jaundice may be detected with ultrasound, particularly if they change the fundamental echotexture of the liver, such as cirrhosis. Obstructive jaundice can be from calculi obstructing the neck of the gallbladder or within the biliary tree or from extrinsic compression on the biliary system, for example a mass at the head of the pancreas, cholangiocarcinoma (tumour within the bile ducts) or a mass compressing the biliary ducts near the porta hepatis. Bilirubin levels may help in the assessment of jaundice and has two forms. It begins as unconjugated (lipid soluble) before being conjugated in the liver, making it water soluble. Abnormal levels of unconjugated bilirubin generally occur if there is an obstruction before the bile gets into the liver, such as non-obstructive causes of jaundice. If the levels of conjugated bile are raised it is often associated with obstructive jaundice, in so much as there is a blockage between the liver and the digestive tract. Careful assessment for obstructive causes is required.

Liver function tests (LFTs) are a group of tests that are used to assess the overall health of the liver and biliary system. They can be used in association with the patient's clinical history, family history and ultrasound findings to assist in reaching a diagnosis. Abnormal tests can give early indications of serious conditions. If the liver is diseased and the cells are damaged, various enzymes will be released into the bloodstream, for example alanine transaminase (ALT) or alkaline phosphatase (ALP).

A short summary is provided below, but further reading around the topic is advised:[3,4]

- ALP is generally raised in non-obstructive jaundice and hepatocellular damage.
- ALT is often raised when there is hepatocellular damage.
- Aspartate aminotransferase (AST) might be raised in both obstructive and non-obstructive hepatobiliary cases.
- Gamma-glutamyl transferase (GGT) often relates to obstructive biliary disease. It can also be increased in alcoholic liver disease and in association with drug-induced liver damage.

It is important to remember that some LFTs can be deranged due to non-hepatobiliary causes, such as AST, which can be found, for example in skeletal muscle, the kidneys and heart muscle.

Other blood tests are also relevant to the hepatobiliary system and include serum albumin, which can be associated with liver disease (low levels, due to the effect the disease can have on the ability of the liver to produce albumin), alpha-fetoprotein, which is sometimes raised in hepatocellular carcinoma, and prothrombin time.

Pancreas: blood tests for amylase and lipase

Amylase is usually present in the blood and urine in small quantities. When cells in the pancreas are injured, as in pancreatitis, or the pancreatic duct is blocked by a gallstone or pancreatic tumour, increased amounts of amylase enter the bloodstream, increasing concentrations in the blood and also in the urine as it is excreted.

Lipase levels are frequently very high in acute pancreatitis, often 5–10 times higher than the highest reference value. Lipase concentrations rise within 24–48 hours of an acute pancreatic attack and may remain elevated for about 5–7 days. Amylase levels tend to rise and fall slightly sooner than lipase levels.

Lipase concentrations may also be raised in pancreatic duct obstruction, pancreatic cancer and other pancreatic diseases; in association with drugs such as codeine, indomethacin and morphine. Moderately increased levels can be linked to other conditions such as kidney disease (due to decreased clearance from the blood), salivary gland inflammation, a bowel obstruction or peptic ulcer disease. Decreased lipase levels may indicate permanent damage to the lipase-producing cells in the pancreas.

THE PANCREAS

Ultrasound is often used as the first-line investigation of the pancreas, as the liver and biliary tree can be assessed at the same time to look for any complications of pancreatic pathology, such as biliary tract dilatation. Additional investigations such as CT, magnetic resonance cholangiopancreatography (MRCP) or endoscopic ultrasound maybe used to complement ultrasound.

Indications

An ultrasound scan of the pancreas and biliary tree is warranted in patients presenting with epigastric pain, nausea and vomiting, jaundice or abnormal blood test results such as increased amylase and lipase, C-reactive protein or abnormal LFTs. Ultrasound of the pancreas is commonly included within a full upper abdominal survey, as there are many complex conditions linking the organs in this region.

Imaging procedure

It is advisable to scan the pancreas at the beginning of the examination before bowel gas rises and obscures the pancreas and epigastric region. With the patient in a supine position on the couch, a curvilinear probe of 2.5–5 MHz is placed in the midline at the level of the xiphisternum. After an initial longitudinal survey of the upper abdomen has been performed (**Figure 2.1**), there often needs to be a slight caudal angle to obtain good views of the pancreas, using the left lobe of the liver as an acoustic window in transverse section (**Figures 2.2** and **2.3**). The pancreas is located superior to the splenic vein (SV) and is located using the landmarks of the SV and superior mesenteric artery (SMA) (see **Figures 2.1** and **2.3**). Often the head and body of the pancreas can be seen more easily than the tail, as in **Figure 2.4**.

The full length of the pancreas is best assessed in a transverse section of the upper abdomen. The shape, size, outline and echotexture of the pancreas are assessed before turning the probe through 90° into a longitudinal section. Slowly sweeping the probe from right to left will demonstrate the pancreas in cross-section from the head to the tail (**Figure 2.1**).

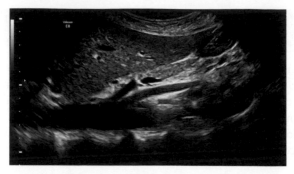

Figure 2.1 A longitudinal section in the epigastric region, showing the anterior branches of the aorta, the coeliac axis (short vessel) and the superior mesenteric artery (longer vessel). Rotation of the probe to a transverse section of the abdomen at this point should bring the pancreas into view.

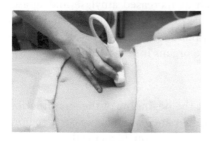

Figure 2.2 Probe positioned for a transverse section of the epigastric region to visualise the pancreas.

Many upper abdominal organs have a capsule, but the pancreas, being a retroperitoneal structure, does not have a capsule, so the outline may be less well defined, and in some cases the pancreas can be challenging to visualise.

There are techniques that can help to overcome this:

- The patient can be asked to push their abdomen towards the transducer.
- The Valsalva breathing technique may be employed.
- Erect scanning may be helpful if the patient is able to sit upright.

If the pancreas is not clearly seen because of overlying bowel gas, the patient can be asked to drink a glass of water, preferably water that has been standing for a little while and has no air bubbles in it. The water fills the stomach and acts as an acoustic window, which can aid visualisation in many cases.[5] Combining water load and erect scanning is often successful.

Image analysis

The normal pancreas is usually comma shaped, with the head being slightly larger than the tail (**Figure 2.3**). In younger patients, the pancreas is slightly darker (hypoechoic) or similar in texture to the liver. With increasing age, the pancreas becomes more fatty and thus becomes brighter in echotexture (hyperechoic). In addition to these age-related changes, acute pancreatic disease will often cause swelling and inflammation, making the pancreas appear hypoechoic on ultrasound, whereas chronic disease will cause fibrosis and shrinkage, making the pancreas appear hyperechoic on ultrasound. The sonographer should observe the pancreas carefully for these changes in echotexture as well as observing the presence of pseudocysts and masses.

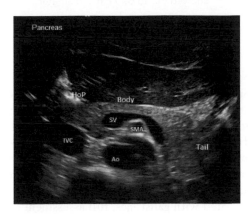

Figure 2.3 Transverse section of the epigastric region demonstrating the pancreas. HoP, head of pancreas; IVC, inferior vena cava; SV, splenic vein; SMA, superior mesenteric artery; Ao, aorta.

The pancreatic duct (PD) is often seen within the pancreas, particularly when the transducer is 90° to the duct (**Figure 2.4**). The PD should measure no more than 2 mm in anteroposterior (AP) diameter. If pathology is found within the pancreas, it is important to check the intra- and extrahepatic bile ducts for dilatation, and the upper abdomen should be assessed for pancreatic pseudocysts in the case of suspected pancreatitis (**Figure 2.5**).

The two main pathologies of the pancreas are pancreatitis and carcinoma. In acute pancreatitis the ultrasound findings may be normal; in other cases the pancreas can appear enlarged and more hypoechoic.

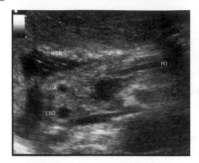

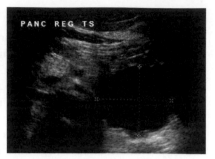

Figure 2.4 Transverse section of the epigastric region demonstrating the common bile duct (CBD) and gastroduodenal artery (GDA) at the head of pancreas (HoP). The pancreatic duct (PD) is also demonstrated.

Figure 2.5 Pancreatic pseudocyst in association with pancreatitis. The electronic measurement callipers showed this to be 7 cm in diameter.

The hypoechoic areas may be focal or diffuse throughout to the whole pancreas. As part of the process of inflammation, pancreatic enzymes often leak into the retroperitoneal space, causing pseudocysts (**Figure 2.5**). These pancreatic pseudocysts are collections of fluid within the retroperitoneum and are often unusual in shape, due to their location within the retroperitoneum. Usually the fluid appears anechoic (black). In chronic inflammation, the pancreas can become coarse in echotexture and may contain areas of calcification (**Figure 2.6**). As pancreatitis is commonly associated with gallstones, full assessment of the gallbladder and biliary tree is an essential part of the examination.

The most common type of pancreatic carcinoma is adenocarcinoma. The majority of cases are located in the head of the pancreas (**Figure 2.7**). Masses are usually hypoechoic, irregular in outline, with increased vascularity demonstrated with colourflow or power Doppler. If the mass is at the head of the pancreas it can cause obstruction, which may lead to dilatation of the PD (dilated if >2 mm), common bile duct (CBD) (dilated if >6 mm, subject to age and other factors), intrahepatic bile ducts and gallbladder. Palpation or sonographic visualisation of an enlarged gallbladder, particularly in the presence of painless jaundice, is known as 'Courvoisier's sign', and is suggestive of a relatively long-standing and progressive obstruction of the bile ducts, in other words more likely to be due to a tumour than to obstruction by a stone.[6]

If a suspicious lesion is found in the pancreas, a thorough investigation of the liver for metastases and the abdomen for ascites and lymphadenopathy is essential. Most patients with suspicious pancreatic lesions are referred for further imaging using CT or MRI, although recent advances in sonography of the pancreas, including endoscopic ultrasound, have overcome some of the issues in imaging this organ.[7]

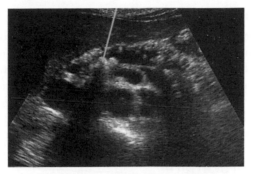

Figure 2.6 Chronic pancreatitis. The pancreas is irregular in outline, the pancreatic duct is dilated and there is calcification within the duct (arrow).

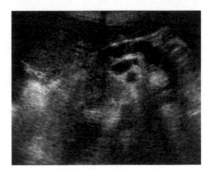

Figure 2.7 Pancreatic adenocarcinoma at the head of pancreas. The pancreatic parenchyma is difficult to see due to dilatation of the pancreatic duct (anechoic), caused by compression due to the tumour. The tumour measures approximately 2.5 cm.

THE LIVER AND BILIARY SYSTEM

The liver and gallbladder are easily accessible by ultrasound and are common areas for referral from both general practice and specialist clinicians. The bile ducts and associated structures can also be assessed during the examination, along with other upper abdominal organs.

Indications

The most common referrals for liver and biliary ultrasound are fatty food intolerance, right upper quadrant (RUQ) pain, deranged LFTs and jaundice. Liver sonography may also be undertaken following discovery of pathology elsewhere in the body to check for metastatic disease or to examine the liver texture, which can be affected by medications for a range of conditions. Follow-up surveillance scans for the assessment of liver disease are common, particularly in cirrhosis or hepatitis.

Imaging procedure

Initially, the patient should lie in the supine position, enabling the sonographer to perform a survey scan beginning with a longitudinal section just under the xiphisternum and gently sweeping from the midline to either side, using a curvilinear probe of 3–7 MHz (**Figure 2.8**). Here the left lobe of the liver can be demonstrated along with the aorta and its associated structures (see **Figure 2.1**) and the right lobe along with the right kidney. A high-frequency linear transducer can be helpful in assessing the anterior liver surface.

The patient should also be scanned in the left posterior oblique position, namely with the right-side half raised, as in **Figure 2.9**, which is very useful for imaging the structures of the biliary system. The lateral decubitus position is often helpful too. Such rotation will alter the position of structures relative to the ribs, making visualisation of the organs easier. Breathing techniques should be adopted to assist further and images are generally frozen on arrested inspiration, which will push the liver down and away from the ribs so that the posterior aspect can be demonstrated. It is vital to use every means possible to ensure that the whole of the liver has been visualised, including intercostal

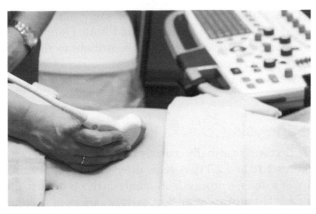

Figure 2.8 With the patient supine, the probe is directed under the rib cage to visualise the superior portion of the liver.

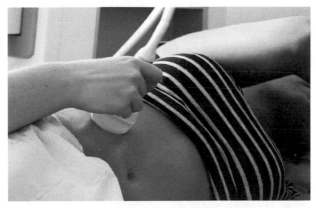

Figure 2.9 The patient is in the left posterior oblique position, which is useful for visualising the liver and biliary system.

and subcostal scanning. Arresting inspiration lessens movement blur to enable assessment of the echotexture and accurate measurements.

Each structure should be imaged in two orthogonal planes to reduce the risk of missing any pathology and eliminate artefact more easily. The size, outline and echotexture of the liver should be examined, along with the outline of the vessels to check for mass effect (deviation of the vessels).

Lesions presenting with a similar echotexture to normal liver tissue (isoechoic) are difficult to delineate, and both Doppler studies and contrast-enhanced ultrasound (CEUS) contribute to the evaluation of liver texture; metastases generally exhibit altered blood flow characteristics, which result in the contrast agent outlining them much more clearly.[8]

Image analysis

Liver echotexture is normally coarsely homogeneous, and of a mid-grey tone (**Figures 2.10** and **2.11**). A generalised brighter appearance may be suggestive of a disease process, commonly cirrhosis or fatty infiltration, whereas focal lesions may represent cysts, a variety of tumours including metastatic disease or other growths. Assessment of smoothness or otherwise in the liver outline will aid in the process; a very uneven outline with surface irregularities or nodularity is suggestive of pathology.[9]

The probe should be directed cephalically to visualise the superior parts of the liver, including the confluence of the hepatic veins with the inferior vena cava (IVC), as in **Figure 2.12**.

Hepatomegaly (enlargement of the liver) is best demonstrated by loss of the sharp edge at the inferior margin of the left lobe (see **Figure 2.10**)

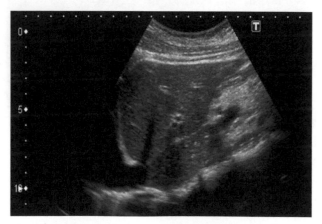

Figure 2.10 A midline sagittal section showing the left lobe of the liver, with a sharp liver edge visible. This is one criterion used to assess for hepatomegaly; an enlarged liver may have a more rounded inferior edge.

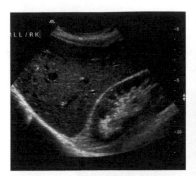

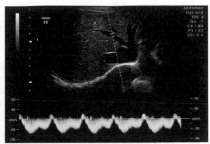

Figure 2.11 The right lobe of the liver in longitudinal section, with the diaphragm visible superiorly. A normal right kidney is also seen; a marked difference in echotexture will alert the sonographer to possible pathology.

Figure 2.12 A transverse section of the liver showing the confluence of the hepatic veins as they drain into the inferior vena cava. This is a duplex scan, showing normal triphasic flow; in diffuse liver disease, flow can be dampened and this triphasic appearance lost.

and right lobe of the liver. Liver measurements can be taken, but these will vary depending on the build of the individual, and guidelines suggest that a reliable and reproducible method of ultrasound measurement has not been established.[10] Therefore, in practice, liver size should always be assessed in conjunction with clinical and other imaging findings as hepatomegaly is generally suggestive of pathology.

Figure 2.13 shows the irregular echotexture characteristic of diffuse metastatic disease throughout the liver. Occasionally a liver sonogram may reveal a solitary metastasis; in such instances, it is helpful for the planning of surgery and other treatment if this can be localised to a particular segment of the liver, known as Couinaud segments. Localisation by ultrasound has been found to be as accurate as MRI.[11]

Neoplastic lesions, particularly in the liver, have variable echogenicity, which is often subtle in nature, and may even be isoechoic, making them very difficult to detect. With the introduction of ultrasound contrast agents, ultrasound can now fully characterise the enhancement pattern of hepatic lesions in a way similar to that achieved with contrast-enhanced multiphasic CT and MRI. CEUS offers high spatial and temporal resolution, and research has reported sensitivities and specificities that rival those of CT and MRI.[12] There are now recommendations for the use of CEUS in best practice guidelines[13,14]

(**Figure 2.14**). This has transformed the identification and characterisation of focal liver lesions and can be of particular help with indeterminate lesions that cannot be diagnosed using other modalities (**Figure 2.15**).

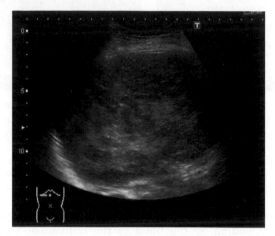

Figure 2.13 Enlarged and heterogeneous liver showing appearances typical of diffuse metastatic disease.

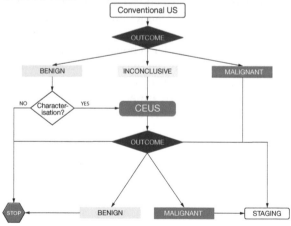

Figure 2.14 Diagnostic pathway for liver imaging with CEUS, as a replacement for contrast-enhanced CT/contrast-enhanced MRI.[13] CEUS, contrast-enhanced ultrasound; CT, computed tomography; MRI, magnetic resonance imaging; US, ultrasound.

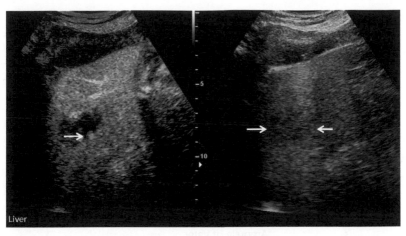

Figure 2.15 A liver haemangioma with contrast (left) compared with the same lesion without contrast (right). The contrast image demonstrates the typical arterial filling pattern of a haemangioma, with peripheral enhancement in the arterial phase.

If a suspicious lesion or a fluid collection is seen during an upper abdominal examination, it may be possible for biopsy or drainage to proceed under ultrasound control. In known chronic liver disease, elastography is now recommended for diagnosis and monitoring of liver changes and may also replace liver biopsy in some cases.[15-17]

If the patient is jaundiced, assessment of the biliary system can distinguish between obstructive and non-obstructive jaundice. **Figure 2.16** shows the gallbladder appearing as a fluid-filled (black) structure, but there are also several white circular areas within the gallbladder representing gallstones, and these inhibit the passage of sound to produce

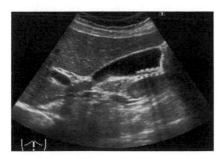

Figure 2.16 A section through the liver showing the gallbladder with stones present; note the strong echoes from the surface of the gallstones and the posterior acoustic shadowing beyond them.

acoustic shadowing beyond. The appearance of gallstones is one of the commonest findings in sonography for epigastric or RUQ pain. Passage of a gallstone into the duct system is one of several possible causes of obstructive jaundice, resulting in dilatation of the biliary tree. This can be demonstrated quantitatively by a measurement of what is known in the ultrasound world as the 'common duct'.

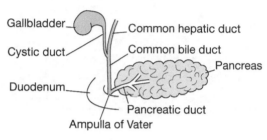

Figure 2.17 The bile duct system.

The bile duct system comprises the left and right hepatic ducts, which join to form the common hepatic duct; this joins the cystic duct leading to and from the gallbladder, and distal to this is the CBD, which passes through the head of the pancreas and drains into the duodenum (**Figure 2.17**). Because the junction between the cystic duct and the common hepatic duct is at an acute angle, it may be difficult to visualise on ultrasound, meaning that it is not always possible to identify the difference between the cystic duct and the CBD with certainty. This has led to the use of the sonographic term common duct, to indicate either of these structures. The standard place to measure the CBD is where the hepatic artery passes anterior to the CBD at the porta hepatis (**Figures 2.18** and **2.19**). A normal common duct measurement in a patient who still has a gallbladder is less than 6 mm, although this can be wider with increasing age over 60 years (approximately 1 mm per decade).

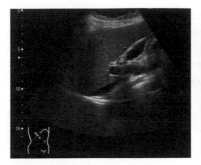

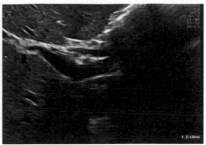

Figure 2.18 A section taken at the porta hepatis, showing the gallbladder and the portal vein, and anterior to this the common duct.

Figure 2.19 When assessing the common duct, the image is magnified to improve visualisation. A measurement greater than 6 mm in an adult suggests possible obstruction and should prompt further evaluation.

THE PORTAL VENOUS SYSTEM

The portal vein is an important vessel for supplying the liver and can be affected by diffuse liver disease such as cirrhosis.

Indications

The portal vein should always be assessed during the routine upper abdominal scan. However, this becomes much more important in patients with known liver disease or in post-transplant recipients.

Following insertion of a transjugular intrahepatic portosystemic shunt (TIPSS), the flow is checked by ultrasound.

Imaging procedure

The portal vein is assessed using B mode, spectral and colourflow Doppler. Using a curvilinear array of 2.5–5 MHz, portal vein measurement and assessment in B mode can be undertaken with the patient in the supine, oblique or decubitus position. Measurement of the portal vein diameter should be taken with the portal vein horizontal across the monitor. The portal vein is assessed for not only for AP diameter, but also for internal echoes, suggestive of thrombosis.[18] Evaluation of the flow within the portal vein is best performed with the patient in the decubitus position with the right-side raised. This allows intercostal scanning from the right side, to ensure a good Doppler angle (<60°). Both spectral and colourflow Doppler should be used to determine the direction of flow within the portal vein. Spectral Doppler can also assess the velocity of flow within the vessel and determine if there is damping of the waveform, associated with disease of the portal venous system.

Image analysis

The portal vein should measure less than 16 mm in AP diameter and should have no internal echoes. The normal spectral Doppler waveform shows forward flow throughout the cardiac cycle with a slightly undulating appearance of the Doppler trace, as in **Figure 2.20**.

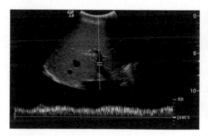

Figure 2.20 Normal B mode and spectral Doppler trace of the portal vein. The trace is taken from within the Doppler gate – the two small parallel lines seen on the B mode image.

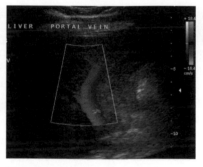

Figure 2.21 Colourflow Doppler appearances of the portal vein showing normal hepatopetal flow.

Colourflow Doppler should show hepatopetal flow, which in **Figure 2.21** is towards the probe. Direction of flow is checked by correlation with the colour scale on the image, which depends on the equipment settings. In this case, the red signal correlates with the top part of the scale seen on the right of the image, indicating flow towards the transducer.

In portal hypertension, commonly found in patients with chronic liver disease such as cirrhosis, there may be reduced flow or even reversed flow in the portal vein. This appears as a lower velocity or a reversal in the spectral Doppler trace, as shown in **Figure 2.22**, by the spectral trace being below the axis; compare with a normal trace in **Figure 2.20**. Colourflow Doppler also demonstrates the direction of flow, in this instance the blue coloration, which is away from the liver, although the scale is omitted from this image. It is vital to ensure that the scale settings are accurate before drawing conclusions about direction of flow.

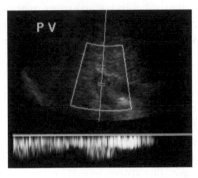

Figure 2.22 Reversed (hepatofugal) flow in the portal vein due to cirrhosis.

Very severe liver disease may cause portal venous thrombosis. This can be treated by an interventional procedure known as TIPSS. This creates a connection directly from the portal vein to one of the hepatic veins, with a stent inserted to retain patency. **Figure 2.23** shows a post-procedure scan, using colourflow Doppler to demonstrate patency.

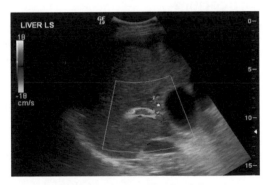

Figure 2.23 Portal venous Doppler following transjugular intrahepatic portosystemic shunt.

THE SPLEEN

The spleen is examined as part of a full upper abdominal ultrasound survey. Focal splenic pathology is uncommon; however, enlargement (splenomegaly) of the spleen is frequently encountered. When scanning the spleen, the diaphragm is usually seen clearly, enabling visualisation of the areas above or below the diaphragm to look for pleural effusions or ascites, respectively. This is especially useful in trauma cases, where a rapid diagnosis is needed to determine the presence of free fluid, to help determine management options.

Indications

Sonography of the spleen is specifically requested in patients with an enlarged palpable spleen on examination, or in cases of unexplained anaemia, fatigue, increased white cell count and infection. Splenomegaly is common in patients with human immunodeficiency virus (HIV) and acquired immune deficiency syndrome (AIDS), portal hypertension and associated liver disease. The spleen would be assessed as part of the overall upper abdominal examination in these cases. A common specific indication for ultrasound of the spleen is in trauma cases, where the clinician needs to know if there is free intra-abdominal fluid or evidence of rupture to the spleen itself.

Imaging procedure

If the patient is in the supine position on the couch, a curvilinear probe of 2–5 MHz is placed against the left side, between the ribs in the intercostal position, to locate the spleen. The spleen is situated superior to the left kidney and can be deceptively high in some cases. If the spleen is difficult to assess in the supine position, turning the patient on to the right side (right lateral decubitus) may help to locate it. This is also better ergonomically for the sonographer, as it avoids stretching across the patient (**Figure 2.24**).

The patient should practise gentle respiration, rather than deep inspiration, during the examination. This is because the diaphragm movement on deep inspiration can cause the spleen to rise further under the ribs.

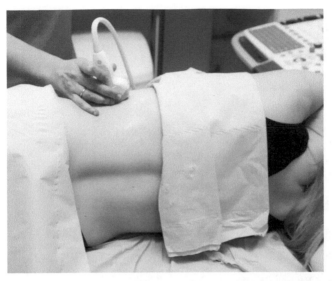

Figure 2.24 Examination of the spleen with the patient in the right lateral decubitus position.

Once the spleen has been located in the longitudinal section, it is important to scan all the way through, looking at the shape, size, outline and echotexture in addition to checking for movement of the diaphragm. A measurement should be taken from the upper to the lower pole of the spleen, to assess the splenic length (**Figures 2.25** and **2.26**). The spleen is also assessed in the transverse section, carefully looking for any focal lesions. Doppler can be used to assess vascularity of focal lesions, or absence of blood flow in trauma or infarcts.

Image analysis

The normal spleen is smooth in outline, with homogeneous mid-grey internal echoes (**Figures 2.25** and **2.26**). The normal length of the spleen is up to 12–13 cm in its long axis. The splenic vessels can often be seen at the splenic hilum.

It is quite common to see a small accessory spleen or splenunculus, appearing as a small, rounded area of splenic tissue (**Figure 2.27**). These can be single or multiple and are insignificant findings, related to the embryological development of the spleen.[19]

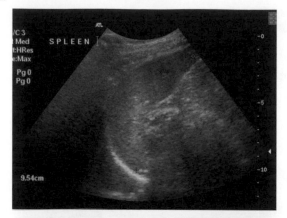

Figure 2.25 A normal spleen. The electronic callipers indicate the overall length to be 9.5 cm, which is within the normal size range.

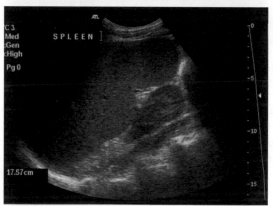

Figure 2.26 Splenomegaly – an enlarged spleen, with an overall length of nearly 18 cm.

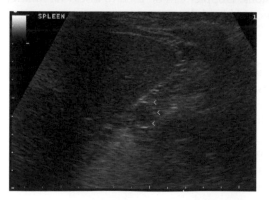

Figure 2.27 A splenunculus, or accessory spleen, seen as a rounded area just below the inferior border. These are relatively common and in some cases may be multiple.

Splenomegaly is evident when the spleen measures more than 13 cm in length (**Figure 2.26**). Note the rounded inferior border on the right of the image, another indicator of enlargement (compare with **Figure 2.25**).

In cases of trauma, particularly in the resuscitation room, it is important to look in the left upper quadrant for free fluid, which can readily be seen with ultrasound (**Figure 2.28**). The spleen itself can also be assessed for focal changes in the echotexture, which may suggest parenchymal damage. Appearances of splenic trauma vary depending on the time of the scan after injury and whether this has been blunt trauma or a penetrating injury, as with stab wounds.[20] Usually there is distortion of the normal smooth homogeneous echotexture, which may be hyperechoic or hypoechoic.

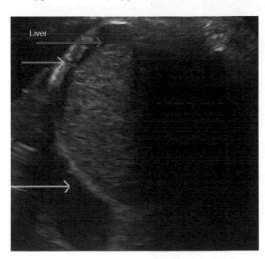

Figure 2.28 A case of blunt abdominal trauma resulting in fluid (red arrow) below the diaphragm (blue arrow) and a pleural effusion above the diaphragm (green arrow).

Focal lesions of the spleen, although uncommon, may be found. Simple cysts appear as anechoic, round, well-defined structures with posterior acoustic enhancement (**Figure 2.29**). In patients with fever and infection, abscesses may be found in the spleen. An abscess is generally heterogeneous (mixed echoes) and may exhibit shadowing from gas within. Ultrasound can be used to guide needle insertion to drain an abscess. It can also be helpful to follow up cases after treatment with antibiotics or following drainage.

Hypoechoic, rounded lesions may be seen in patients with lymphoma (**Figure 2.30**) or could potentially be secondary metastases from a primary tumour elsewhere, particularly gynaecological tumours of ovarian origin, breast, lung and colorectal carcinomas. A hyperechoic lesion could indicate a haemangioma, which has a similar appearance to a haemangioma in the liver. A wedge-shaped hypoechoic lesion within the spleen, with no evidence of blood flow demonstrable with colour-flow or power Doppler, may be suggestive of a splenic infarct.

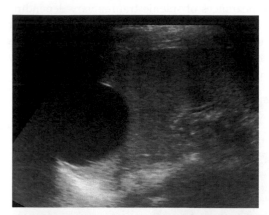

Figure 2.29
A simple splenic cyst demonstrating good through transmission of the sound with no internal echoes, and acoustic enhancement seen beyond.

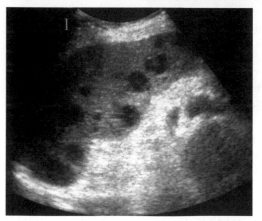

Figure 2.30 Spleen exhibiting lesions typical of lymphoma.

REFERENCES

1. Ehrenstein BP, Froh S, Schlottmann K, Schölmerich J, Schacherer D. To eat or not to eat? Effect of fasting prior to abdominal sonography examinations on the quality of imaging under routine conditions: A randomized, examiner-blinded trial. *Scandinavian Journal of Gastroenterology.* 2009:**44**(9);1048–1054. doi: 10.1080/00365520903075188.
2. Bellamy EA, Bossi MC, Cosgrove DO. Ultrasound demonstration of changes in the normal portal venous system following a meal. *British Journal of Radiology* 1984;**57**(674);147–149. doi: 0.1259/0007-1285-57-674-147.
3. Hall P, Cash J. What is the real function of the liver 'function' tests? *Ulster Medical Journal* 2012;**81**(1):30–36. PMID: 23536736.
4. Giannini EG, Testa R, Savarino V. Liver enzyme alteration: A guide for clinicians. *Canadian Medical Association Journal* 2005;**172**(3):367–379. doi: 10.1503/cmaj.1040752.
5. MacMahon H, Bowie JD, Beezhold C. Erect scanning of pancreas using a gastric window. *American Journal of Roentgenology* 1979;**132**(4): 587–591. doi: 10.2214/ajr.132.4.587.
6. Fitzgerald JE, White MJ, Lobo DN. Courvoisier's gallbladder: Law or sign? *World Journal of Surgery* 2009;**33**(4):886–891. doi: 10.1007/s00268-008-9908-y.
7. Dimcevski G, Erchinger FG, Havre R, Gilja OH. Ultrasonography in diagnosing chronic pancreatitis: New aspects. *World Journal of Gastroenterology* 2013;**19**(42):7247–7257. doi: 10.3748/wjg.v19.i42.7247.
8. D'Onofrio M, Crosara S, De Robertis R, Canestrini S, Mucelli RP. Contrast-enhanced ultrasound of focal liver lesions. *American Journal of Roentgenology* 2015;**205**(1):W56–W66. doi: 10.2214/AJR.14.14203.
9. Yeom SK, Lee CH, Cha SH, Park CM. Prediction of liver cirrhosis, using diagnostic imaging tools. *World Journal of Hepatology* 2015;**7**(17);2069–2079. doi: 10.4254/wjh.v7.i17.2069.
10. Dietrich CF, Serra C, Jedrzejczyk M. Ultrasound of the liver. EFSUMB – European course book, 2010. Available at: http://issuu.com/efsumb/docs/coursebook-ultrasoundliver_ch02?e=3336122/6603908
11. Conlon RM, Bates JA. *Segmental localisation of focal hepatic lesions – a comparison of ultrasound and MRI.* Conference proceedings of the British Medical Ultrasound Society, Edinburgh 1996. Cited in Smith JA. *Abdominal ultrasound: How, why and when*, 3rd edn. London: Churchill Livingstone, 2010.

12. Morin SH, Lim AKP, Cobbold JFL, Taylor-Robinson SD. Use of second generation contrast-enhanced ultrasound in the assessment of focal liver lesions. *World Journal of Gastroenterology* 2007;**13**(45); 5963–5970. doi: 10.3748/wjg.v13.45.5963.

13. NICE (National Institute for Health and Care Excellence). *SonoVue (sulphur hexafluoride microbubbles) – contrast agent for contrast-enhanced ultrasound imaging of the liver. Diagnostics guidance [DG5],* 2012. Available at: https://www.nice.org.uk/Guidance/dg5.

14. Nolsøe CP, Lorentzen T. International guidelines for contrast-enhanced ultrasonography: Ultrasound imaging in the new millennium. *Ultrasonography* 2016;**35**(2):89–103. doi: 10.14366/usg.15057.

15. Barr RG, Ferraioli G, Palmeri ML, Goodman ZD, Garcia-Tsao G, Rubin J, et al. Elastography assessment of liver fibrosis: Society of Radiologists in Ultrasound Consensus conference statement. *Radiology* 2015;**276**(3);845–861. doi: 10.1148/radiol.2015150619.

16. NICE (National Institute for Health and Care Excellence). *Hepatitis B (chronic): Diagnosis and management of chronic hepatitis B in children, young people and adults. Clinical guideline [CG165],* 2017. Available at: https://www.nice.org.uk/guidance/cg165.

17. NICE (National Institute for Health and Care Excellence). *Virtual touch quantification to diagnose and monitor liver fibrosis in chronic hepatitis B and C. Medical technologies guidance [MTG27],* 2020. Available at: https://www.nice.org.uk/guidance/mtg27.

18. Khan AN, Al-Khattab Y, Tam C-L, Sheen AJ. Portal vein thrombosis imaging. Medscape, 2018. Available at: http://emedicine.medscape.com/article/373009-overview.

19. Yildiz AE, Ariyurek MO, Karcaaltincaba M. Splenic anomalies of shape, size, and location: Pictorial essay. *The Scientific World Journal* 2013;321810. doi: 10.1155/2013/321810.

20. Lupien C, Sauerbrei EE. Healing in the traumatized spleen: Sonographic investigation. *Radiology* 1984;**151**(1).181–185. doi: 10.1148/radiology.151.1.6701312.

Further reading

Dietrich C, Bamber J, Berzigotti A, Bota S, Cantisani V, Castera L, et al. EFSUMB guidelines and recommendations on the clinical use of liver ultrasound elastography, update 2017 (long version). *Ultraschall in der Medizin* 2017;**38**(4):e16–e47. doi: 10.1055/a-0641-0076.

Dietrich CF, Nolsøe CP, Barr RG, Berzigotti A, Burns PN, Cantisani V, et al. Guidelines and good clinical practice recommendations for contrast enhanced ultrasound (CEUS) in the liver – update 2020 – WFUMB in cooperation with EFSUMB, AFSUMB, AIUM, and FLAUS. *Ultraschall in der Medizin* 2020;**41**(5):562–585. doi: 10.1055/a-1177-0530.

SIMTICS. *Ultrasound training: spleen.* SIMTICS sonography e-learning suite. Uploaded 19 Dec 2010. YouTube. Available at: http://www.youtube.com/watch?v=xigBZjS8aog.

CHAPTER 3
THE RENAL TRACT

The kidneys   68
The urinary bladder   78
References   84

THE KIDNEYS

Ultrasound has widely superseded intravenous urography as the imaging modality of choice for the renal system because of its ready availability and ease of application, as well as there being no risks from ionising radiation or iodinated contrast media.

The kidneys are particularly amenable to sonography because of their superficial location, and because renal disease is often characterised by changes in the size, shape and echotexture of the kidneys, all of which can be readily seen by ultrasound. The ureters are not normally visualised, except when dilated.

Several blood tests can assess renal function. Creatinine is a metabolic waste product, which is excreted from the blood plasma by the kidneys, and a raised serum creatinine (SCr) level indicates impaired renal function, normal levels being typically in the range of 0.5–1.2 mg/dl. The estimated glomerular filtration rate (eGFR) takes into account variables such as age, sex and SCr levels. Levels of greater than 90 ml/min per 1.73 m^2 are considered normal. Levels below this value indicate impaired renal function.

Indications

Renal ultrasound is indicated in cases of loin pain, haematuria, abnormal kidney function tests, screening for the familial condition of polycystic kidneys and in babies and children to follow up antenatally detected conditions such as pyelectasis (dilated renal pelvis). It is used to monitor known kidney disease, to monitor the health of transplanted kidneys and to guide biopsy procedures.

Patient preparation

No special preparation is necessary to scan the kidneys, although there is the opportunity to examine the other upper abdominal organs if the patient is fasted, and certainly the renal arteries are more easily identifiable.

Bladder filling may be indicated with certain renal symptoms in order to examine the bladder for tumours, stones or other conditions.

In this case, the patient should take a pint and a half of water (or other clear fluid) an hour before the examination. Over-filling of the bladder may cause dilatation of the renal pelvises, giving a false impression of hydronephrosis; if this is suspected, the kidneys should be re-scanned 15 minutes post-micturition.

Imaging procedure

Using a curvilinear probe of 2.5–5 MHz, the kidneys should be scanned on arrested inspiration in order to move them down from under the rib cage and temporarily immobilise them. The patient's arm should be raised above the head to lift the lower costal margin and open up the intercostal spaces. As with all structures, the kidneys must be scanned in both longitudinal and transverse sections. A true longitudinal section is essential for measuring bipolar length. Coronal sections are best to display the pelvicalyceal systems, ureter and main blood vessels.

The long axis of the right kidney is usually best seen with the patient in the left prone oblique position, using the liver as an 'acoustic window' (**Figure 3.1**). It may be necessary to scan intercostally to see the upper pole and subcostally for the lower pole. It can be difficult to see the left kidney in a sagittal section as it is often obscured by the stomach and the splenic flexure of the colon, and so a supine approach is not recommended. It is best scanned in the right lateral decubitus position, with a coronal approach (**Figure 3.2**). This also minimises risk of sonographer strain, as attempts at scanning the left kidney with the patient supine

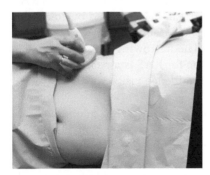

Figure 3.1 Suggested position for assessing the right kidney.

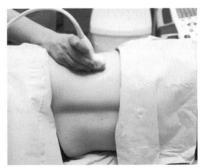

Figure 3.2 Suggested position for assessing the left kidney.

require over-stretching on the part of the sonographer. The spleen can be used as an acoustic window for the upper pole, whereas the more posterior approach shown may be necessary for the lower pole.

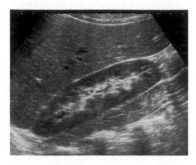 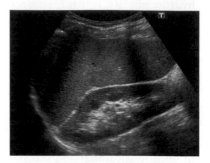

Figure 3.3 A longitudinal section of the right kidney: normal appearance. The liver, as well as serving as an 'acoustic window', can be used as a comparator for the echotexture of the kidney.

Figure 3.4 A longitudinal section of the left kidney: normal appearance. The renal capsule, some of the pyramidal system and the brighter area of the fatty central renal sinus are clearly seen.

Image analysis

Normal kidneys appear regular in shape and have a smooth outline (**Figures 3.3** and **3.4**). They should be seen in real time to move easily with respiration. The kidneys in any individual are normally found to be of roughly equal size, with the normal renal length around 9–12 cm. If the renal lengths differ by more than 2 cm, renal artery stenosis (RAS) may be suspected.[1] The renal arteries can be identified by colourflow Doppler, and spectral Doppler is used to observe the waveform and measure the peak systolic velocity. The narrowing causes an increase in velocity and the diagnostic criterion for RAS is a peak systolic velocity of more than 200 cm/s,[2] with turbulence visible in the waveform beyond this.

The kidney parenchyma is normally about 2.0–2.5 cm thick, and should be of similar echogenicity to liver, as shown in **Figure 3.3**. Chronic renal disease results in smaller, fibrotic kidneys that appear relatively brighter on ultrasound, with thinner parenchyma.[3] The parenchyma also atrophies with age,[4] so that in elderly people the kidneys may show similar appearances. The renal pyramids may be seen as hypoechoic triangular areas between the cortex and the sinus, shown best in **Figure 3.4**. The pyramids are generally more prominent in neonates and younger patients.

The renal sinus normally appears hyperechoic, as in **Figures 3.3** and **3.4**, because of the fat surrounding the vessels. The sinus contains the calyces and the renal pelvis, but these structures are not usually seen unless they are dilated. Ultrasound has a high sensitivity and specificity for the detection of obstructive conditions of the kidneys, but small kidney stones may be difficult to see, although any measuring 2 mm or more should be readily detectable. Reverberation demonstrated on colourflow Doppler, when it is known as 'twinkle artefact', can be helpful in diagnosing small renal calculi, as can using a narrow field of view (**Figure 3.5**).

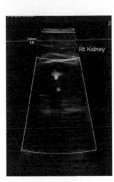

Figure 3.5 A narrow field of view and colourflow Doppler can assist in visualisation of small renal calculi.

It is important to be aware of common anatomical variants, which are frequently seen within the kidney, such as:

- extrarenal pelvis, which is just outside the kidney and commonly seen in the transverse section (**Figure 3.6**);
- splenic (dromedary) hump on the left kidney; a slight bulge usually at the mid-point of the left kidney – note the difference in shape between the kidneys in **Figures 3.3** and **3.4**;
- hypertrophied column of Bertin, in which the cortex of the kidney extends into the renal sinus at the mid-point;
- fetal lobulation, which is seen as small indentations into the otherwise smooth renal outline;
- duplex kidney, containing two collecting systems. The kidney is usually larger than expected and two separate collecting

systems can be seen (**Figure 3.7**), particularly when scanning in longitudinal section;

- ectopic kidney: this is when one or both kidneys are located away from the renal fossa, most commonly in the pelvis. If the kidney is not seen when scanning, check the pelvis carefully.

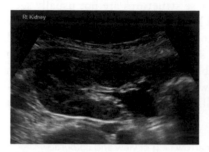

Figure 3.6 A transverse section of the right kidney showing an extrarenal pelvis, visible as the fluid area beyond the renal outline.

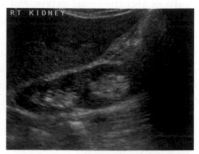

Figure 3.7 A duplex right kidney, with two collecting systems.

Many kidney conditions are connected with developmental anomalies,[5] and so these are seen relatively frequently. The embryological development of the kidney is recommended study for a better understanding of these anomalies.

Renal cysts are easily detectable; an example is shown in **Figure 3.8**. These are very common and of no clinical significance in the absence of symptoms and if they have no internal structure. A renal cyst with internal content should be investigated further and, although computed tomography (CT) scanning has long been the gold standard for

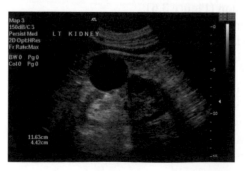

Figure 3.8 A 'simple' renal cyst arising from the parenchyma, the signature appearance being that there is no internal content.

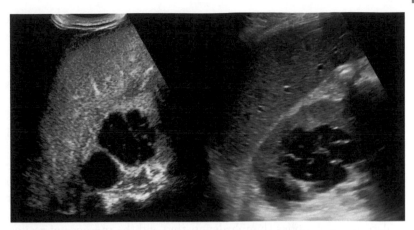

Figure 3.9 Contrast-enhanced ultrasound (left) of a complex renal cyst (arrowed), compared with the baseline image (right). The contrast image shows no enhancement of the echogenic areas within the cyst, suggesting a low chance of malignancy.[7]

staging of complex renal cystic masses using the Bosniak classification, recent studies are showing excellent results with contrast-enhanced ultrasound (CEUS) (**Figure 3.9**).[6]

In the case of polycystic kidney disease, both kidneys generally contain multiple cysts of varying sizes, with renal enlargement and loss of clear renal outline (**Figure 3.10**). Clinically, with this hereditary disease, patients usually present between 30 and 40 years of age with

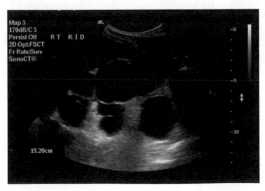

Figure 3.10 Right kidney, with a polycystic appearance.

a range of symptoms such as reduced renal function, loin and flank pain and possibly haematuria. It can often be difficult to measure the bipolar length of an enlarged kidney accurately (**Figure 3.10**), and in this instance the report should state 'measures in excess of 15 cm'. It is important to assess other organs such as the liver and spleen for cysts when polycystic kidneys are suspected or diagnosed.

Solid lesions are shown in **Figures 3.11** and **3.12**. **Figure 3.11** shows a heterogeneous (solid, mixed echo) mass, which is likely to be a renal tumour. This appearance is common in renal cell carcinoma (RCC). Patients with renal tumours often present in the late stages of the disease process with haematuria and/or loin pain. It is important to assess for spread of a renal tumour into the renal vein and inferior vena cava, in addition to other areas of spread such as liver metastases, enlarged lymph nodes (lymphadenopathy) and the presence of ascites. **Figure 3.12** demonstrates a small hyperechoic mass at the upper pole of the right kidney. This is most likely to be an angiomyolipoma; the high fat content gives this characteristic bright appearance. Colourflow and power Doppler can investigate any suspected renal masses. CEUS may also play a role in the differentiating solid lesions.[8]

Renal vein thrombosis may occur in cases of nephritic syndrome and is a potential complication of renal tumours, although the vast majority of cases occur in neonates. Ultrasound is a rapid and non-invasive way of investigating this condition.

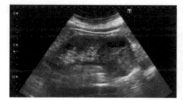

Figure 3.11 A solid lesion at the lower pole of the left kidney (to the right of the image).

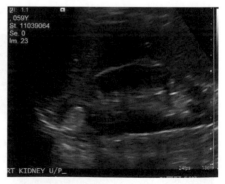

Figure 3.12 A hyperechoic angiomyolipoma at the upper pole of the right kidney (to the left of the image).

Hydronephrosis, or fluid accumulation within the renal collecting system, is a common finding when scanning the kidneys (**Figure 3.13**). Ultrasound is useful to determine the cause of an obstruction that can lead to hydronephrosis, to assess the severity of obstruction and for follow-up examinations after treatment, such as lithotripsy. Some centres use a grading system to define the severity of hydronephrosis and this consists of assessing whether the dilatation affects the renal pelvis alone or includes slight calyceal dilatation, with or without blunting of the calyces, and whether there is associated cortical thinning. Causes of hydronephrosis can include tumours and calculi anywhere within the renal tract, strictures such as at the pelvi-ureteric junction (PUJ; also known as the uteropelvic junction or UPJ) causing obstruction, or an enlarged prostate or pregnancy pushing on the urethra or ureters.

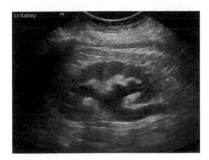

Figure 3.13 Slight hydronephrosis and hydroureter, with normal cortical thickness.

Hydronephrosis can also be seen in urinary tract infections (UTIs). In severe cases, pus can collect in the urinary tract, causing pyonephrosis, which appears as internal echoes within the fluid. Additional findings with UTIs include focal or diffuse changes in echotexture and reduced vascularity of the parenchyma in pyelonephritis. In chronic cases, cortical thinning and/or cortical scarring can be seen. Cortical scarring is differentiated from fetal lobulation (a normal variant) by looking for a hyperechoic linear structure indenting the renal outline and extending to the renal sinus (**Figure 3.14**).

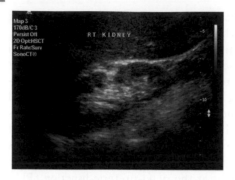

Figure 3.14 Renal scarring in a case of long-standing chronic urinary tract infection. RT, right.

PUJ obstruction is a congenital abnormality of the urinary tract, which is caused by a stricture at this junction. It is more common in males and can cause an appearance similar to hydronephrosis, and indeed is often identified as hydronephrosis on antenatal ultrasound. The differentiating feature of PUJ obstruction is that the upper ureter does not appear dilated (**Figure 3.15**), whereas a true hydronephrosis will also show dilatation of the upper ureter (**Figure 3.13**). Spectral Doppler studies to evaluate resistive index (RI) values and ratios may also be used as a differentiating factor.[9]

Nephrocalcinosis is caused by calcium deposits within the kidney (**Figure 3.16**). Patients may be asymptomatic but can present with symptoms such as UTIs or renal calculi. There may be a history of hyperparathyroidism. The calcium deposits are commonly in the medullary region but can be in the cortex. In medullary nephrocalcinosis, the medullary pyramids are hyperechoic instead of having their normal

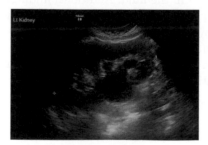

Figure 3.15 Pelvi-ureteric junction obstruction. Lt, left.

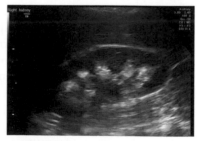

Figure 3.16 Nephrocalcinosis; hyperechoic renal pyramids.

anechoic appearance. In some patients, there may be acoustic shadowing, but this is not always the case.

Ultrasound can be useful in assessing patients following renal transplantation. The kidney is transplanted into the pelvis and is susceptible to a range of complications. Ultrasound is used to monitor patients due to the ease of repeatability and being non-ionising. Early pelvicalyceal dilatation can be easily detected, as can vascular complications and fluid collections. Biopsy under ultrasound guidance can be used to determine whether there is rejection of the transplant kidney and ultrasound can be used to assist with drainage of fluid collections. An initial ultrasound examination is used as a baseline postoperatively, to allow comparison for further follow-up examinations. The transplant kidney is superficially located in the pelvis, enabling the use of a high-frequency transducer for best resolution. Power Doppler is useful to check perfusion in a transplant kidney.

The ultrasound examination of a transplant kidney should assess:

■ renal echogenicity – changes could indicate inflammation, infection, infarct, although they are non-specific;
■ renal size, to check for changes in renal volume;
■ pelvicalyceal dilatation;
■ renal artery and vein for signs of thrombus;
■ fluid collections around the transplant kidney, which may represent haematoma, urinoma, abscess or lymphocele. A small amount of free fluid is common postoperatively.

Signs of rejection of the transplant kidney include enlarged renal pyramids, increased renal size, the presence of oedema, reduced cortico-medullary differentiation and changes to flow rates within the renal artery.[10]

THE URINARY BLADDER

As a fluid-filled structure, the urinary bladder is amenable to ultrasonic imaging. Ultrasound is particularly acceptable in children, where bladder conditions may be common, and is useful for dynamic studies.

Indications

Indications for bladder ultrasound include pain, dysfunction and haematuria, although ultrasound has shown poor sensitivity in comparison with cystoscopy for the latter.[11] Abdominal and pelvic trauma, whether blunt injury or fractures, may damage the bladder, which is also susceptible to penetrating injuries. Prenatally detected or chronic conditions may be followed up.

The role of ultrasound in the assessment of the older male patient with lower urinary tract symptoms is to assess:

- bladder wall thickness and appearances;
- prostate size;
- post-micturition bladder residue;
- hydronephrosis in the kidneys – common in cases of an enlarged prostate.

Patient preparation

Sonography of the bladder requires filling as outlined in the introduction. A filled volume of 350–500 ml is usually sufficient to perform the investigation. Under-filling may not allow for complete imaging of the bladder, whereas over-filling may cause a false appearance of hydronephrosis if the kidneys are to be examined at the same time. The best course of action is to scan the bladder and then ask the patient to void if the examination is to include the kidneys as well.

If the patient is catheterised, check that the catheter can be clamped off and fluid given an hour prior to the investigation. Infection control is particularly important if the patient is catheterised.

In cases of suspected urinary retention, the patient should not be asked to fill their bladder until retention has been excluded by a preliminary scan.

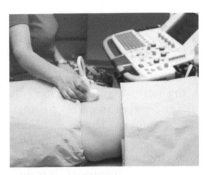

Figure 3.17 Probe positioned for a longitudinal section of the bladder.

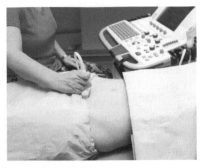

Figure 3.18 Probe positioned for a transverse section of the bladder.

Figure 3.19 Longitudinal section of a bladder with a diverticulum.

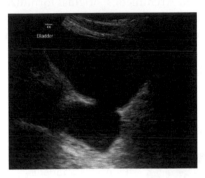

Imaging procedure

The bladder is scanned in longitudinal and transverse sections (**Figures 3.17** and **3.18**) using a curvilinear probe of 2.5–5 MHz. Positive identification of the bladder must be made, because ovarian cysts and other discrete fluid areas may be mistaken for the bladder, just as large diverticula of the bladder may be mistaken for ovarian cysts or other cystic pathology (**Figure 3.19**). The lower ureters may be seen by scanning obliquely at the area of the trigone, angling the probe laterally, with the ureteric orifices appearing as small, thickened areas.

Image analysis

On longitudinal scans the full bladder may appear almost triangular, whereas on transverse scans it may appear virtually oblong (**Figure 3.20**).

Dimensions may be measured to calculate the bladder volume (**Figure 3.20**). This is not useful in the normal full bladder, as the capacity is too variable to establish norms, except in cases of urinary retention and in children with nocturnal enuresis. However, bladder volume can be used for quantifying any post-micturition residue. Almost all equipment now includes an automatic volume calculator, into which the sonographer need only enter the dimensions. It is difficult to know exactly what formulae individual manufacturers use, but they are generally likely to be based on Archimedes' original formulae for calculating the volume of a sphere ($V = 4/3.\pi.r^3$). If it is necessary to calculate this manually, the technique originally described by Poston et al.[12] may be used:

$$\text{Volume (in ml)} = 0.7 \times H \times D \times W$$

where H = maximum diameter in the longitudinal plane, D = depth in the longitudinal plane and W = maximum width in the transverse plane, with all measurements taken in centimetres.

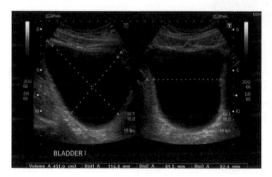

Figure 3.20 The normal full bladder in longitudinal section (left) and transverse section (right).

In the example of **Figure 3.20**, the machine calculation is seen to be 451 cm³ whereas using Poston's formula the measurements (which have to be converted into centimetres) would yield 598 cm³. This demonstrates the variability of calculations. The most reliable means of measuring bladder volume is by three-dimensional ultrasound,[13] although this may not be readily available in many urology or general ultrasound facilities. However, the key point to remember in calculating volume is that the purpose of this is to be able to indicate if there is a significant residue, which is likely to give rise to infection, rather than to produce an absolute and accurate figure.

The bladder wall and contents must be examined. The wall should be of smooth outline, with no filling defects or protuberances, and with a thickness of about 2–3 mm in the full bladder and up to 5 mm in the post-micturition bladder.

It is common to see diverticulae (**Figure 3.19**) and thickening of the urinary bladder wall (**Figure 3.21**), particularly in patients with urinary retention.

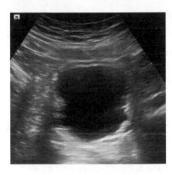

Figure 3.21 Transverse section of a bladder with a thickened wall.

The motion of urinary jets emanating from the ureteric orifices into the bladder can often be seen in real time on greyscale imaging. Identification of the ureteric orifices can be useful to exclude a localised bladder wall thickening at this point. They have been enhanced by the use of colourflow Doppler for illustrative purposes in **Figure 3.22**.

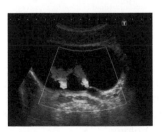

Figure 3.22 The normal full bladder in transverse section, with ureteric jets visible at the base of the bladder.

The bladder contents should be clear, with no debris or other content. It is important to ensure that the time gain compensation and gain settings are optimised to reduce artefact (**Figure 3.23**), which might otherwise be confused with debris (**Figure 3.24**). Bladder debris can often be seen to move with patient movement.

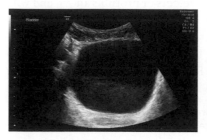 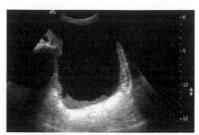

Figure 3.23 Suboptimal equipment settings, which can be mistaken for debris within the bladder.

Figure 3.24 Shows bladder debris, visible as echoes in the posterior aspect of the urinary bladder.

Bladder calculi have the same appearance as calculi in other areas; they are generally mobile and hyperechoic with posterior shadowing (**Figure 3.25**). In the renal tract, calculi often cause haematuria.

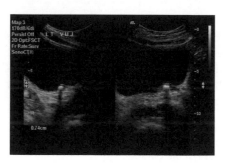

Figure 3.25 Bladder calculi, with acoustic shadowing. LT VUJ = left vesico ureteric junction.

Haematuria may also be caused by urothelial carcinoma, and differentiation between bladder calculus and bladder tumour is an important role of ultrasound. **Figure 3.26** shows a tumour in an 88-year-old man who presented with haematuria. Cystoscopy may be needed for further assessment of tumours and other bladder pathology.

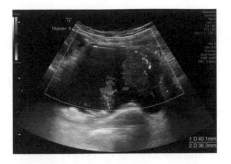

Figure 3.26 Urothelial carcinoma, previously called transitional cell carcinoma.

Other abnormal bladder findings may include polyps and even foreign bodies.

The prostate may be visualised in the adult male as a rounded hypo-echoic structure at the base of the bladder. An enlarged prostate gland indenting the bladder is not uncommon in older men. Prostatic enlargement can lead to a range of symptoms such as frequency of micturition, nocturia, dribbling, often collectively known as lower urinary tract symptoms (LUTS). Causes for enlargement of the prostate include prostatitis, benign prostatic hypertrophy (BPH) and prostate cancer. Ultrasound findings should be reviewed in relation to other investigations, such as prostate-specific antigen (PSA) blood test results. PSA can be raised in association with prostate cancer. The prostate can be assessed in more detail using transrectal ultrasound, using a dedicated high-frequency probe. This gives higher resolution images, and can be used to guide prostate biopsy, as described in Chapter 4 on 'The male reproductive system'. The normal prostate is said to measure less than 30 ml, and a technique for transrectal ultrasound prostate volume measurements has been documented.[14] Other methods of assessment include Doppler, elastography, CEUS multi-parametric dynamic CEUS, and fusion imaging with MRI.[15,16] Ultrasound guidance can be used to ensure accurate placement of radioactive 'seeds' for brachytherapy in patients with prostate cancer.

REFERENCES

1. Granata A, Fiorini F, Andrulli S, Logias F, Gallieni M, Romano G, et al. Doppler ultrasound and renal artery stenosis: An overview. *Journal of Ultrasound.* 2009;**12**(4):133–143. doi: 10.1016/j.jus.2009.09.006.

2. Williams GJ, Macaskill P, Chan SF, Karplus TE, Yung W, Hodson EM, et al. Comparative accuracy of renal duplex sonographic parameters in the diagnosis of renal artery stenosis: Paired and unpaired analysis. *American Journal of Roentgenology* 2007;**188**(3):798–811. doi: 10.2214/AJR.06.0355.

3. Ozmen CA, Akin D, Bilek SU, Bayrak AH, Senturk S, Nazaroglu H. Ultrasound as a diagnostic tool to differentiate acute from chronic renal failure. *Clinical Nephrology* 2010;**74**(1):46–52. PMID: 20557866.

4. Emamian SA, Nielsen MB, Pedersen JF, Ytte L. Kidney dimensions at sonography: Correlation with age, sex, and habitus in 665 adult volunteers. *American Journal of Roentgenology* 1993;**160**(1):83–86. doi: 10.2214/ajr.160.1.8416654.

5. Schedl A. Renal abnormalities and their developmental origin. *Nature Reviews Genetics* 2007;**8**(10):791–802. doi: 10.1038/nrg2205.

6. Girometti R, Stocca T, Serena E, Granata A, Bertolotto M. Impact of contrast-enhanced ultrasound in patients with renal function impairment. *World Journal of Radiology* 2017;**9**(1):10–16. doi: 10.4329/wjr.v9.i1.10.

7. Nicolau C, Bunesch L, Sebastia C. Renal complex cysts in adults: Contrast-enhanced ultrasound. *Abdominal Imaging* 2011;**36**(6):742–752. doi: 10.1007/s00261-011-9727-8.

8. Ignee A, Straub B, Brix D, Schuessler G, Ott M, Dietrich C. The value of contrast enhanced ultrasound (CEUS) in the characterisation of patients with renal masses. *Clinical hemorheology and microcirculation* 2010;**46**(4):275–290. doi: 10.3233/CH-2010-1352. Corpus ID: 24621624

9. Riahinezhad M, Sarrami AH, Gheisari A, Shafaat O, Merikhi A, Karami M, et al. How may Doppler indices help in the differentiation of obstructive from nonobstructive hydronephrosis? *Journal of Research in Medical Sciences* 2018;**23**:76. doi: 10.4103/jrms.JRMS_627_17.

10. Sutherland T, Temple F, Chang S, Hennessy WK, Lee W-K. Sonographic evaluation of renal transplant complications: Renal transplant ultrasound. *Journal of Medical Imaging and Radiation Oncology* 2010;**54**(3):211–218. doi: 10.1111/j.1754-9485.2010.02161.x.

11. Purnell VE, Desai S, Husain J, Dodgeon J. Is bladder ultrasound indicated as part of the routine investigation of haematuria? *Ultrasound* 2011;**19**(4):209–213. doi: 10.1258%2Fult.2011.011012.

12. Poston GJ, Joseph AE, Riddle PR. The accuracy of ultrasound in the measurement of changes in bladder volume. *British Journal of Urology* 1983;**55**(4):361–363. doi: 10.1111/j.1464-410x.1983.tb03322.x.

13. Ghani KR, Pilcher J, Rowland D, Patel U, Nassiri D, Anson K. Portable ultrasonography and bladder volume accuracy – a comparative study using three-dimensional ultrasonography. *Urology* 2008;**72**(1):24–8. doi: 10.1016/j.urology.2008.02.033.

14. Aprikian S, Luz M, Brimo F, Scarlata E, Hamel L, Cury FL, et al. Improving ultrasound-based prostate volume estimation. *BMC Urology* 2019;**19**(1):68. doi: .10.1186/s12894-019-0492-2.

15. Mitterberger M, Horninger W, Aigner F, Pinggera GM, Steppan I, Rehder P, et al. Ultrasound of the prostate. *Cancer Imaging* 2010;**10**(1): 40–48. doi: 10.1102/1470-7330.2010.0004.

16. Wildeboer RR, Postema AW, Demi L, Kuenen M, Wijkstra H, Mischi M. Multiparametric dynamic contrast-enhanced ultrasound imaging of prostate cancer. *European Radiology* 2017;**27**(8):3226–3234. doi: 10.1007/s00330-016-4693-8.

CHAPTER 4

THE MALE REPRODUCTIVE SYSTEM

Transrectal ultrasound (TRUS) of the prostate gland   88
The scrotum and testes   92
The penis   103
References   105

TRANSRECTAL ULTRASOUND (TRUS) OF THE PROSTATE GLAND

Although some information on the prostate may be obtained during a transabdominal examination of the prostate gland, using the bladder as an acoustic window (**Figure 4.1**), dedicated imaging is more usually performed by a transrectal examination, whereby an endocavity probe is inserted into the rectum as a means of directly imaging the prostate. This is shown diagrammatically in the section on 'Prostatic biopsy' (p. 92).

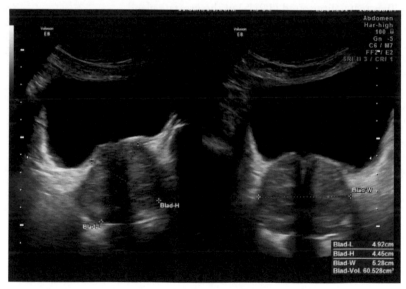

Figure 4.1 Transabdominal images of the prostate gland. The volume function has been used to measure and calculate prostatic volume.

Indications

TRUS may be indicated if there have been abnormal blood test results, for example raised prostate-specific antigen (PSA), which is produced by the prostate gland and is the key screening test for early detection of prostate cancer. A level of 3–4.0 ng/ml or below is considered normal. Although a raised level may indicate the presence of prostate cancer, the test can be misleading; some men with raised levels of PSA may not have cancer and those with normal levels may actually have the disease. TRUS is also used as a guide for prostate biopsy for definitive diagnosis.[1]

Patient preparation

No physical preparation is required for the direct visualisation of the male reproductive organs other than the removal of clothing below the waist. It is of course important to consider the privacy and dignity of the patient throughout, and consider the potential of a chaperone, as in all intimate examinations.

A slightly distended urinary bladder is useful in imaging the base of the prostate via a transabdominal scan.

Although uncomfortable, TRUS is a relatively painless procedure carried out after an initial clinical digital rectal examination. A cleansing enema may be necessary if there is a great deal of faecal material in the rectum.

If the examination is to proceed to biopsy, local anaesthetic is required.

Imaging procedure

There are two types of transrectal probe, known as 'side-fire' and 'end-fire', which relate to the siting of the crystals that form the transducer face. Those probes with crystals at the end will produce a sector-shaped image similar in shape to the transvaginal probe images, and the plane of this image is dependent on the direction in which the probe is angled, so this technique is more likely to be used in the lithotomy position to enable greater manoeuvrability of the probe. Probes with crystals arranged peripherally around the shaft of the probe will produce a circular image in which the central black area represents the probe position. This will yield sequential axial sections of the anatomy as the probe is advanced.

Because of the nature of the examination, cross-contamination is relatively easy. To prevent this, the probe must be disinfected immediately before and after use. Gloves must be worn by the sonographer.

Best practice guidelines for decontamination of the probe and machine should be followed, using manufacturer-approved processes.[2]

To ensure good image quality, all air must be removed from the probe assembly. A dedicated probe cover is used with gel inside and sterile ultrasound coupling gel is then applied to the tip of the covered probe.

For TRUS, the patient generally lies on his left side with the knees drawn up to enable probe insertion with the minimum risk to rectal tissues, although the lithotomy position may also be used with care.

Measurements are taken, enabling calculation of the overall volume of the prostate. If it is thought to be enlarged, or if a discrete lesion is identified, a biopsy is possible if the patient consents, to retrieve tissue to be sent for histology to diagnose or exclude prostate cancer in the tissue sample.

Image analysis

All the transrectal images (**Figures 4.2**, **4.3** and **4.4**) utilise an 'end-fire' probe, so the sections are coronal, with the top of the image representing the more superior anatomy, and the black semicircle at the bottom of the image representing the probe position at the base of the rectum.

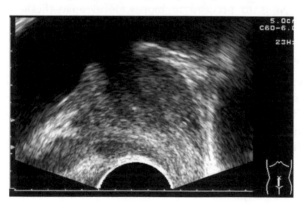

Figure 4.2
A transrectal sonogram of a normal prostate gland of homogeneous echotexture.

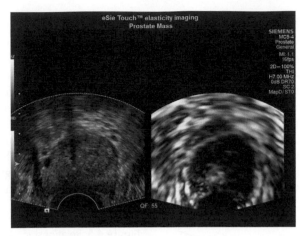

Figure 4.3 A similar section to **Figure 4.2**, but there is a prostatic mass demonstrated in the near field. The two images are B mode (left) and greyscale elastography (right). The elastography image on the right displays the relative stiffness of tissue as calculated from the returning echoes, and clearly demonstrates the mass.

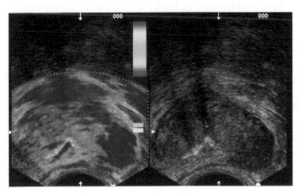

Figure 4.4 A prostatic mass, demonstrated on the left using a colour map of tissue texture obtained by elastography. The mass is blue, suggesting 'hard' tissue, which is more likely to be malignant in nature.

Prostatic biopsy

There are two biopsy approaches: transrectal biopsy and transperineal biopsy.[3] Bleeding can occur during transrectal biopsy and this may lead to sepsis, so a course of prophylactic broad-spectrum antibiotics is prescribed for 1 week prior to biopsy. The risk of infection is greatly reduced in transperineal biopsy. Local anaesthetic should be infiltrated into the periprostatic region for a transperineal biopsy.[4]

In both approaches, cores of tissue are obtained through an 18-gauge biopsy needle. For transrectal biopsy, the needle is attached to an automatic trigger device and directed by ultrasound (**Figure 4.5**). For transperineal biopsy, the needle may be placed through a special guiding device attached to the transducer.

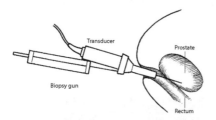

Figure 4.5 Relationship of a biopsy needle and the prostate gland in the transrectal approach.

THE SCROTUM AND TESTES

The scrotum lies below the symphysis pubis, in front of the upper parts of the thighs and behind the penis. It contains the testes, the epididymides and lower spermatic cords (**Figure 4.6**).

Ultrasound imaging of the scrotum is fairly commonly deployed, since it is the primary imaging method used to evaluate disorders of the testicles and surrounding areas and can help determine the cause of testicular pain or swelling.

Indications

Pain or swelling in the scrotum, a palpable mass, or history of trauma to the scrotal area can lead to a referral for a scrotal ultrasound examination.[5] Patients undergoing fertility investigations may also have a scrotal ultrasound.

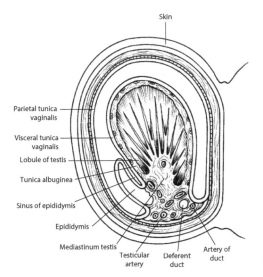

Skin

Parietal tunica vaginalis

Visceral tunica vaginalis

Lobule of testis

Tunica albuginea

Sinus of epididymis

Epididymis

Mediastinum testis

Testicular artery

Deferent duct

Artery of duct

Figure 4.6
Diagram of the scrotum showing internal structures.

A sudden onset of acute scrotal pain requires immediate attention. The most common cause of scrotal pain is epididymitis, treatable with antibiotics. Left untreated, this condition can lead to an abscess or loss of blood supply to the testicles. Another cause for severe pain, which can be detected by ultrasound is testicular torsion – snared twisting of the spermatic cord, which contains the vessels that supply blood to the scrotum. Torsion requires immediate surgery to avoid permanent damage to the testes.

Ultrasound has an important role in the location and evaluation of masses within the male reproductive system. The majority of scrotal masses are sited outside of the testes and are mostly benign, for example an epididymal cyst. A mass sited inside the testicles is more likely to be malignant.

Scrotal ultrasound can also identify a hydrocele, abnormal blood vessels, microlithiasis and scrotal hernia, where some abdominal contents herniate into the scrotum. Ultrasound can also detect an absent or undescended testicle; in rare cases, a testicle may fail to develop, but, more often, it has failed to descend. It is estimated that approximately 3–5% of full-term baby boys have undescended testicles.[6] It is important to diagnose these because there is a very high probability of future infertility and testicular cancer if left untreated.[7]

Patient preparation

The previous notes on privacy and dignity apply, and the patient lies supine or semi-recumbent on the imaging couch. A disposable towel is placed as a 'band' or 'sling' across the thighs and behind the scrotum, to help support and present the scrotum at a suitable aspect for examination, and the patient is usually asked to hold his penis supero-laterally away from the scrotal area. For patient dignity, the area superior to the scrotum may then be covered with a drape, and a blanket placed over the patient's legs.

Imaging procedure

Ultrasound gel is applied to the scrotal skin and a linear array transducer of 7.5–15 MHz is glided gently over the scrotum to perform the examination. In the case of extreme scrotal enlargement, a lower frequency may be required.

The aim is to examine the entire scrotum and its contents in at least two planes (sagittal and transverse). Using real-time B mode, the unaffected hemiscrotum is examined first, using a systematic and sequential scanning action to visualise the area in at least two planes. This provides a reference for comparison with the affected side, which is next examined in a similar manner. A coronal scan that shows both testicles side by side is then performed to allow identification of differences in size and structure (**Figure 4.7**). Throughout the examination, the size, position and echotexture of the relevant structures are assessed. Testicular measurements should be recorded in three planes if there is a marked difference in size. The normal testis measures up to 5 cm × 4 cm × 3 cm. Measurements of any masses or fluid collections are also recorded.

Colourflow Doppler may be useful in the identification of neovascularisation associated with testicular carcinoma. Power Doppler enables assessment of testicular blood flow patterns (**Figure 4.9**), for example, a marked increase in testicular blood flow plus a (reactive) hydrocele indicates orchitis. Power Doppler may be combined with spectral Doppler to identify whether the flow is venous or arterial. Multi-parametric imaging, using a combination of Doppler, contrast-enhanced ultrasound and elastography, can be useful in assessing scrotal pathology.[8]

Image analysis

The normal testes appear homogeneous in texture on ultrasound and should be imaged together for comparison, as in **Figure 4.7**, where they appear of similar echotexture to each other, with a mid-grey appearance.

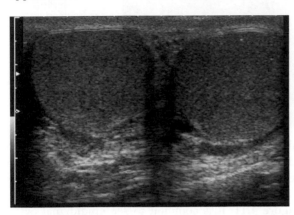

Figure 4.7
A transverse section of both testicles side by side, showing normal appearances.

If extended field-of-view technology is available, this is useful for imaging larger testes or masses (**Figure 4.8**). This enables visual comparison of the size and echotexture of the whole of both testicles, which can help to identify diffuse change. In this case the echotexture is normal.

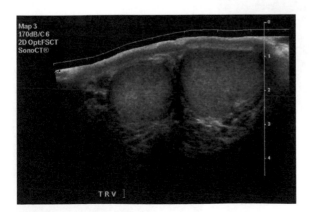

Figure 4.8
A transverse section of the scrotum, using extended field of view, demonstrating the full extent of the testicles.

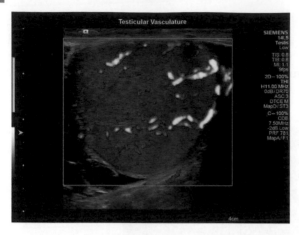

Figure 4.9
Power Doppler demonstrates normal testicular vasculature. Colourflow and power Doppler can be used in the assessment of normal testes and to interrogate focal lesions.

Common normal appearances when scanning the testes include a hyperechoic band of tissue seen across the middle of the testis in **Figure 4.10**, representing the mediastinum testis and the rete testis or spermatic tubules, seen as small anechoic structures close to the mediastinum testis in **Figure 4.11**. It is common to see epididymal cysts, which are often located in the head of the epididymis (**Figure 4.12**).

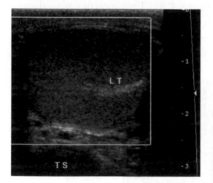

Figure 4.10 (left) Mediastinum testis.

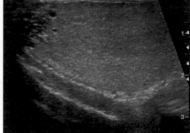

Figure 4.11 (right) The near field contains both the rete testis and a small intratesticular cyst.

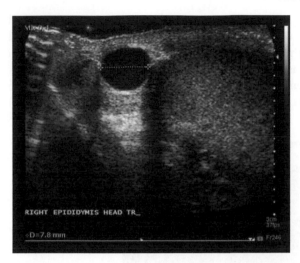

Figure 4.12
A fluid-filled area in the near field is demonstrated and measured at the head of the testis. This is an epididymal cyst, a benign condition seen frequently when scanning the scrotum and requiring no treatment.

Infection within the scrotum can be secondary to urinary tract infection, prostatic pathology or sexually transmitted infection such as chlamydia or gonorrhoea, leading to inflammation within the epididymis (epididymitis). This can spread into the testis, causing orchitis; both conditions together are epididymo-orchitis. The ultrasound appearances include enlargement of the epididymis, which can be focal or diffuse, and hypoechoic appearances of the epididymis and/or the testis (**Figure 4.13**), with increased vascularity on colour-flow Doppler. There can be associated scrotal wall thickening and hydrocele formation.

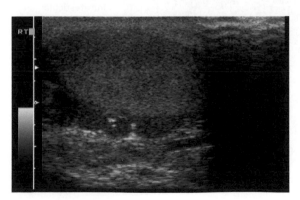

Figure 4.13
Enlarged, hyperechoic epididymis in epididymitis.

Hydroceles are the commonest reason for testicular swelling and are a fairly frequent finding on ultrasound.[9] They are formed by fluid collecting within the tunica vaginalis (see **Figure 4.6**). They may form for no apparent reason (idiopathic) or can be associated with epididymo-orchitis, torsion, tumour or in trauma cases. **Figures 4.14** and **4.15** show hydroceles as a collection of fluid (appearing anechoic or black) around the testis.

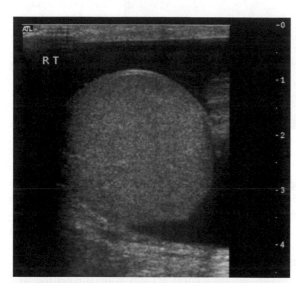

Figure 4.14
Testicular hydrocele.

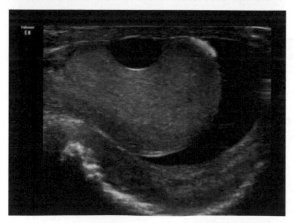

Figure 4.15
Intratesticular simple cyst and a hydrocele.

Intrascrotal masses can be seen readily on ultrasound. It has always been suggested that an intratesticular mass should be presumed malignant until proven otherwise. A number of different methods may be needed to help classify the lesion as benign or malignant. Patients often present with a palpable mass on examination. Incidental intratesticular lesions can be seen during ultrasound examinations for other clinical indications.[10]

Benign intratesticular lesions include:

- Simple cysts, which have the typical sonographic features of a cyst, being rounded, smooth in outline, anechoic with posterior acoustic enhancement and avascular (**Figure 4.15**).
- Epidermoid cysts, which appear as concentric rings of hyper- and hypoechoic echoes: some authors liken it to onion ring or onion skin appearance.[10,11] An example is shown in **Figure 4.16**.
- Abscess – these can vary in appearance, but are generally hypoechoic and may have internal low-level echoes and appear heterogeneous. There can be associated reactive hydrocele, scrotal thickening and possibly gas within the abscess or scrotal cavity.
- Tubular ectasia is a cystic lesion of the rete testis with multiple tubular cystic areas seen in the region of the mediastinum; commonly seen in association with epididymal cysts.

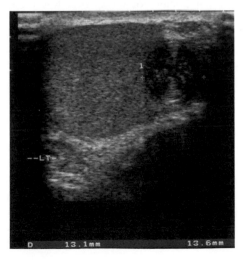

Figure 4.16 Epidermoid cyst.

Solid intratesticular lesions are often germ-cell tumours and may be a seminoma or a non-seminomatous tumour. Seminomas are the most common germ-cell tumours and are often unilateral hypoechoic lesions, as in **Figure 4.17**. Non-seminomatous germ-cell tumours include choriocarcinoma, embryonal cell carcinoma, yolk-sac tumour and teratoma. All have slightly different appearances, but are commonly heterogeneous, with varying degrees of haemorrhage, calcification and/or necrosis. Serum markers of human chorionic gonadotrophin (hCG) and alpha-fetoprotein (AFP) may also be raised.

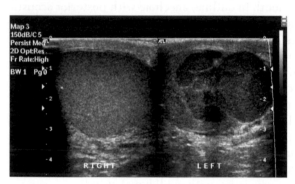

Figure 4.17
A hypoechoic (darker) lesion within the left testis, clearly seen in comparison to the normal right testis. This represents a seminoma.

The treatment and prognosis varies depending on tumour type and stage of detection.[11] The European Society of Urogenital Radiology (ESUR) guidelines on non-palpable testicular lesions suggest that those measuring less than 5 mm should have short-term follow-up, whereas lesions more than 5 mm, such as that in **Figure 4.17**, should undergo partial orchiectomy.[10] It is important to take accurate measurements, particularly for those patients who will be attending for follow-up scans.

Testicular microlithiasis, or microcalcification, is visible as tiny hyperechoic (bright) areas throughout the testicular tissue (**Figure 4.18**). This condition may be associated with various chromosomal aberrations or possibly with testicular cancer. There has been much debate in the literature about the role testicular microlithiasis has in relation to the prediction of testicular cancer. The ESUR guidelines state that, in patients with no associated risk factors, testicular microlithiasis needs no further follow-up or investigations.[12] Patients are advised to undertake monthly self-examination. Annual surveillance is recommended for all patients with associated risk factors, including previous germ-cell tumour, history of maldescent or orchidopexy (surgery to remove an undescended testicle), testicular atrophy or a first-degree relative with a history of germ-cell tumour.

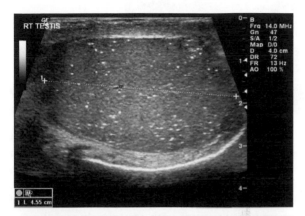

Figure 4.18
Testicular
microlithiasis.

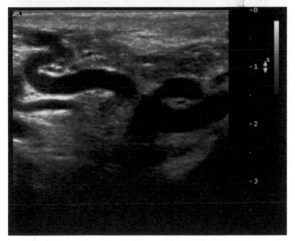

Figure 4.19 Dilated
veins in a testicular
varicocele.

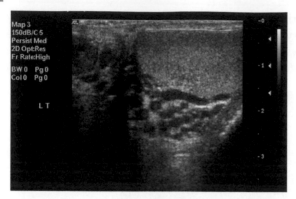

Figure 4.20
Testicular varicocele demonstrated in relation to the left testis.

Varicoceles are a common finding during ultrasound of the scrotum **(Figures 4.19 and 4.20)**. These are dilated veins in the pampiniform plexus, which can be diagnosed clinically, although ultrasound is often requested for confirmation. Varicoceles are more common on the left side, due to the difference in venous drainage. They can be associated with male subfertility and may present with scrotal pain, swelling or a palpable mass. Ultrasound diagnosis is generally suggested when the veins measure 3 mm or more.[13] Suggested technique and standardised reporting are available within the ESUR guidelines.[13] Colourflow Doppler can be used to assess the vessels for reverse flow whereas the Valsalva technique is used to distend the veins.

There is controversy within the literature about whether the kidneys should be assessed when a varicocele has been detected. One review article suggests that in patients under the age of 40 years the chance of an incidental varicocele being caused by a renal tumour was very low.[14] The authors also indicate that, in a patient over 40 with no symptoms other than a varicocele, the chance of having a renal tumour is still low. Conversely, in children under 9 years of age, when varicoceles are not usually seen, there is a higher chance of a varicocele being linked to a Wilms' tumour. A systematic review found that limited research was available to make evidence-based decisions, so the examination should be extended to include the renal tract until further evidence becomes available.[15]

THE PENIS

Indications

Penile ultrasound may be used to investigate strictures, stones or diverticulae in the penile urethra, cases of penile fracture and other trauma, and masses. However, its most common application is in cases of erectile dysfunction (ED), where it may be used to evaluate blood flow.

Patient preparation

The foregoing paragraphs on the preparation for ultrasound examination of the male reproductive system apply.

Imaging procedure

Penile ultrasound is best performed with a high-frequency linear array transducer with an ultrasound frequency of 7.5–18 MHz. As with other ultrasound examinations, penile ultrasound should start with a survey scan comprising both transverse and longitudinal views of the penis to determine the depth of the cavernosal arteries and to evaluate for plaques, intracavernosal lesions and urethral pathology. The goal is to visualise the cross-sectional view of the two corpora cavernosa dorsally and the corpus spongiosum ventrally along the length of the penis, from the base of the penile shaft to the glans penis.[16]

Ultrasound evaluation of penile blood flow in cases of ED involves injecting a vasodilator into the vessels at the base of the penis to induce an erection. Transverse and longitudinal sections of the corpora cavernosa and the corpus spongiosum are once again obtained, and the blood flow observed using Doppler ultrasound to check afferent and efferent flow, to determine whether the dysfunction is due to inflow or outflow causes. The patient should remain in the department until penile detumescence has occurred.

Image analysis

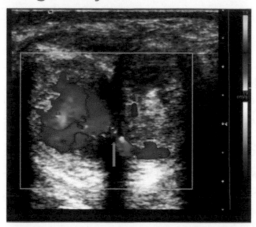

Figure 4.21
An arteriovenous (AV) fistula, which in this case has developed following trauma to the penis. The blue arrow marks (centre) the point of fistulation to a venous lake that has formed within the corpora cavernosa.

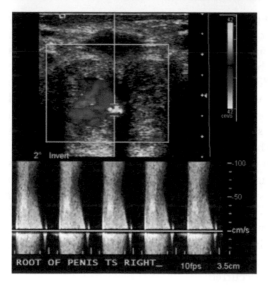

Figure 4.22 Shows a triplex image of the same case. The spectral Doppler trace with the Doppler gate positioned at the point of fistulation shows a high-velocity jet of flow. This can be seen in the colourflow Doppler image as a point of aliasing, where the trace has moved into the opposite channel; the point of maximum velocity appears in green.

Arteriovenous (AV) fistulae can be demonstrated with colourflow and spectral Doppler, as demonstrated in **Figures 4.21** and **4.22**. Priapism is a prolonged penile erection, which may be related to trauma, underlying medical conditions or some pharmaceuticals, among other causative factors. It is painful or at least uncomfortable, and is considered a medical emergency requiring immediate treatment to avoid long-term dysfunction and irreversible infarction. The blue arrows in **Figure 4.23** outline a region of hypoechoic change within the corpora cavernosa, and no blood flow was detected here with colourflow Doppler.

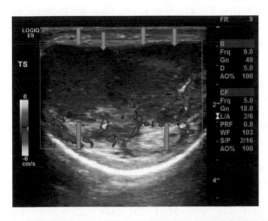

Figure 4.23 Infarction of the penis post-priapism.

REFERENCES

1. Harvey CJ, Pilcher J, Richenberg J, Patel U, Frauscher F. Applications of transrectal ultrasound in prostate cancer. *British Journal of Radiology* 2012;**85**(Suppl 1):S3–S17. doi: 10.1259/bjr/56357549.
2. AXREM, BMUS & SCoR. *Ultrasound transducer decontamination – best practice summary*, 2020. Available at: https://www.axrem.org.uk/resource/ultrasound-transducer-decontamination-best-practice-summary/.
3. Guo LH, Wu R, Xu HX, Xu JM, Wu J, Wang S, et al. Comparison between ultrasound guided transperineal and transrectal prostate biopsy: A prospective, randomized, and controlled trial. *Scientific Reports* 2015;**5**:16089. doi: 10.1038/srep16089.
4. Shetty S. *Transrectal ultrasound of the prostate*. Medscape, 2016. Available at: http://emedicine.medscape.com/article/457757-overview#showall.
5. Kühn AL, Scortegagna E, Nowitzki KM, Kim YH. Ultrasonography of the scrotum in adults. *Ultrasonography* 2016;**35**(3):180–197. doi: 10.14366/usg.15075.

6. Berkowitz GS, Lapinski RH, Dolgin SE, Gazella JG, Bodian CA, Holzman IR. Prevalence and natural history of cryptorchidism. *Pediatrics* 1993;**92**(1):44–49. PMID: 8100060.

7. Hutson JM, Balic A, Nation T, Southwell B. Cryptorchidism. *Seminars in Pediatric Surgery* 2010;**19**(3):215–224. doi: 10.1053/j.sempedsurg.2010.04.001.

8. Auer T, De Zordo T, Dejaco C, Gruber L, Pichler R, Jaschke W, et al. Value of multiparametric US in the assessment of intra-testicular lesions. *Radiology* 2017;**285**(2):640–649. doi: 10.1148/radiol.2017161373.

9. Adhikari S. Testicular Ultrasound. In: Ma J, Reardon R and Joing S (eds), *Emergency Ultrasound*. McGraw Hill Publishers, New York, USA, 2013, 3rd edn, 353–379.

10. Rocher L, Ramchandani P, Belfield J, Bertolotto M, Derchi L, Correas J, et al. Incidentally detected non-palpable testicular tumours in adults at scrotal ultrasound: Impact of radiological findings on management radiologic review and recommendations of the ESUR scrotal imaging subcommittee. *European Radiology* 2016;**26**(7):2268–2278. doi: 10.1007/s00330-015-4059-7.

11. Appelbaum L, Gaitini D, Dogra VS. Scrotal ultrasound in adults. *Seminars in Ultrasound, CT, and MRI* 2013;**34**(3):257–273. doi: 10.1053/j.sult.2013.01.008.

12. Richenberg J, Belfield J, Ramchandani P, Rocher L, Freeman S, Tsili AC, et al. Testicular microlithiasis imaging and follow-up: Guidelines of the ESUR scrotal imaging subcommittee. *European Radiology* 2015;**25**(2):323–330. doi: 10.1007/s00330-014-3437-x.

13. Freeman S, Bertolotto M, Richenberg J, Belfield J, Dogra V, Huang DY, et al. Ultrasound evaluation of varicoceles: Guidelines and recommendations of the European Society of Urogenital Radiology Scrotal and Penile Imaging Working Group (ESUR-SPIWG) for detection, classification, and grading. *European Radiology*. 2020;**30**(1):11–25. doi: 10.1007/s00330-019-06280-y.

14. El-Saeity NS, Sidhu PS. "Scrotal varicocele, exclude a renal tumour". Is this evidence based? *Clinical Radiology* 2006;**61**(7):593–599. doi: 10.1016/j.crad.2006.02.011.

15. Robson J, Wolstenhulme S, Knapp P. Is there a co-association between renal or retroperitoneal tumours and scrotal varicoceles? A systematic review. *Ultrasound* 2012;**20**(4):182–191. doi: 10.1258/ult.2012.012020.

16. Rais-Bahrami S, Gilbert BR. Penile ultrasound. In: Gilbert BR, (ed.), *Ultrasound of the male genitalia*. New York: Springer Science + Business Media, 2015:125–155.

CHAPTER 5
THE GASTROINTESTINAL (GI) TRACT

The salivary glands   108
The adult GI tract   112
Endoscopic ultrasound (EUS)   117
The neonatal GI tract   121
References   124

THE SALIVARY GLANDS

There are three main pairs of salivary glands: the parotid, submandibular and sublingual. The parotid and submandibular glands are triangular and located in the retromandibular fossa and under the body of the mandible, respectively. The sublingual gland lies deep to the mylohyoid muscle, which forms the floor of the mouth. As the salivary glands are superficial structures, they are amenable to high-frequency, high-resolution ultrasound imaging.

Ultrasound is the first-line modality for assessment of the salivary glands as it is safe, non-invasive and well tolerated.[1] It is useful for differential diagnosis of disease of the salivary glands as it can assess the size and echotexture to identify a calculus or other mass, determine the nature of a lesion, confirm or exclude neovascularisation and assess any duct dilatation. It can also be used to guide fine-needle aspiration biopsy or core biopsy for histology or cytology of a lesion.

In some cases, it is not possible to visualise the gland or lesion by ultrasound alone if it extends to the deep lobe of the parotid gland or is obscured by the acoustic shadow of the mandible. In these cases, and in lesions with features suggestive of malignancy, further imaging using computed tomography (CT) or magnetic resonance imaging (MRI) can evaluate deeper structures and the extent of any infiltration.[2]

Indications

Ultrasound of the salivary glands is indicated for the following reasons:
- A palpable lump in the gland or neck.
- Mouth dryness.
- Pain in the glands.
- The patient can sometimes feel a stone under the mandible or under their tongue. A stone can block the duct causing infection and swelling.
- Mumps or other illness, including mouth or dental infections.
- Abnormality on sialogram or other imaging.
- Guidance of injection, aspiration or biopsy.
- Monitoring Sjögren's syndrome for lymphoma development.

Patient preparation

Following explanation of the ultrasound procedure, the patient is asked to loosen and remove clothing and any jewellery from the neck. Paper towels are placed across the chest and shoulders to avoid soiling clothing with coupling gel.

The patient should lie in the supine position, either with a pillow under the shoulders, as shown in **Figure 5.1**, or without a pillow, as in **Figure 5.2**, so that the neck is extended. Coupling gel is applied to the neck to aid transmission of the ultrasound beam.

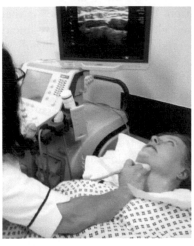

Figure 5.1 (left) Submental approach for scanning the sublingual and submandibular salivary glands.

Figure 5.2 (right) Positioning for scanning the submandibular salivary gland.

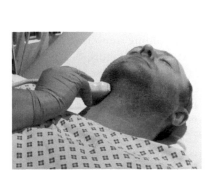

Imaging procedure

Using a 10–12.5 MHz linear array transducer, each entire gland is evaluated in at least 2 perpendicular planes: longitudinal and transverse. The submental approach is used for the sublingual and submandibular glands (**Figure 5.1**), and a more lateral approach for the submandibular gland (**Figure 5.2**). The parotid gland is superior and posterior to this. The head may be turned a little to the opposite side for better lateral access.

B mode images are obtained initially to assess the size of the gland, its echotexture and presence of a lesion. The ducts are assessed for presence of calculus and any dilatation. Colourflow Doppler is then used to assess vascularity within the gland and any lesions found. Transoral ultrasound can also assist in the detection of pathology.[3]

The salivary gland on the opposite side is also scanned for comparison and the whole of the neck examined on both sides to assess the surrounding anatomy, including the cervical lymph nodes.

On completion of the examination the gel is removed, the transducer is cleaned and the results are discussed with the patient or they are given information about obtaining the results from the referrer.

The report on the findings should include documentation of any lesion, including the shape, size, outline, echotexture and vascularity.

Image analysis

The salivary glands normally appear on ultrasound imaging as homogeneous structures with variable echogenicity compared with the surrounding muscles, depending on the amount of intraglandular fatty tissue. **Figure 5.3** illustrates the normal ultrasound features of the submandibular gland; it is triangular with slightly brighter (hyperechoic) parenchyma compared with the surrounding muscles. Normal non-dilated ducts are not visible on ultrasound. The facial artery and vein are located posterior to or within the gland as shown in **Figure 5.4**.

Calculi are found mainly in the submandibular gland rather than the other salivary glands.[4] The ultrasound features of calculi are strong hyperechoic lines or points with distal acoustic shadowing, as shown in **Figure 5.5**. It is important to demonstrate the location of a calculus

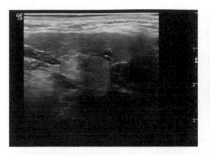

Figure 5.3 Ultrasound image of a normal submandibular gland. Note the generally homogeneous echotexture.

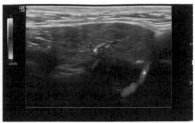

Figure 5.4 Ultrasound image of a normal submandibular gland. The colourflow Doppler overlay displays the arterial perfusion of the gland and the facial artery posteriorly.

as this determines the choice of treatment; there are many pitfalls in salivary gland scanning and care should be taken to distinguish the anatomical structures.[5] In **Figure 5.5**, the calculus appears to be in the parenchyma and no duct dilatation is demonstrated. A dilated duct would be demonstrated as a tubular hypoechoic vessel and should be confirmed by use of colourflow Doppler to differentiate it from a blood vessel.

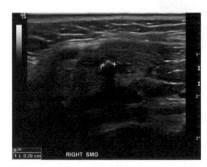

Figure 5.5 A 28mm hyperechoic calculus (measured), with distal acoustic shadowing, is demonstrated within a swollen submandibular gland.

Ultrasound can demonstrate masses in the salivary glands and distinguish between cystic and solid masses. Cysts are well defined and anechoic (no internal echoes), with posterior acoustic enhancement and absence of internal vascularity. Solid lesions are generally well defined, with internal echoes and little or no posterior acoustic enhancement.

The majority of solid lesions are tumours of the salivary glands and tend to be benign as demonstrated in **Figures 5.6** and **5.7**.

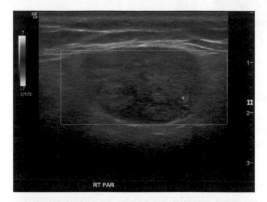

Figure 5.6 Ultrasound of the parotid gland, showing a well-circumscribed, solid, hypoechoic mass within the gland. There is some slight posterior acoustic enhancement and no calcification demonstrated within the mass. The colourflow Doppler overlay shows some internal vascularity.

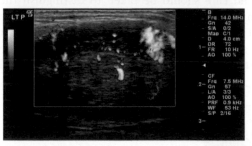

Figure 5.7 Power Doppler better demonstrates low-velocity vascularity.

THE ADULT GI TRACT

Ultrasound is often used as the first-line imaging modality in the investigation of abdominal pain and non-specific GI symptoms. Familiarity with the ultrasound appearances of bowel pathologies is important to achieve the correct diagnosis in symptomatic patients and to allow appropriate triage of patients for further management.

Indications

Ultrasound has a specific role in the following conditions:

- Evaluation of right iliac fossa (RIF) pain to diagnose acute appendicitis.
- Diagnosis of pyloric stenosis and intussusception – although this is more common in children.
- Investigation in neonates of necrotising enterocolitis (NEC), which is described separately in this chapter in the section on 'The neonatal GI tract'.
- Screening, evaluation and detection of abdominal complications and postoperative follow-up of patients with Crohn's disease.

Imaging procedure

The bowel is usually assessed after examining the solid abdominal organs. A tight radius curvilinear probe is used to provide good access via a small contact point, as there may be transmission difficulties due to bowel content or adipose tissue. The highest possible frequency commensurate with adequate penetration should be selected, usually between 4 and 7 MHz based on the body habitus. This frequency provides a good overview of the GI tract and is often sufficient for diagnostic imaging, although subsequently a higher-frequency (7–13 MHz) linear probe may be used; this provides higher-resolution images but has a limited depth of penetration.

A clinical history should be obtained directly from the patient while simultaneously assessing the contents of the abdomen and pelvis, and sonography, thus, becomes an extension of the clinical examination and can be tailored according to the clinical context.

The examination begins in the RIF by identifying the caecum as a blind-ending loop of large bowel, usually in the right lower quadrant. The scan proceeds systematically along the entire length of the colon until the rectosigmoid region is reached in the pelvis. The right lower quadrant is then assessed to identify the appendix and terminal ileum. This is followed by several general sweeps craniocaudally to cover the entire abdomen and pelvis to assess the small bowel loops (**Figure 5.8**).

Graded compression should be applied when scanning the bowel. Normal bowel is readily compressible, shows peristaltic activity and has movable intra-luminal gas; in contrast thickened abnormal bowel is usually rigid and remains unchanged. Assessment using power Doppler and contrast-enhanced ultrasound (CEUS) may demonstrate

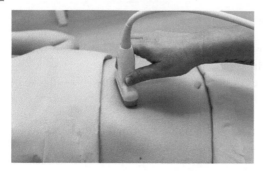

Figure 5.8 The ultrasound probe positioned on the upper abdomen, in this instance for investigation of the proximal small bowel.

increased blood flow to thickened bowel segments, which would support a diagnosis of an acute inflammatory process. These adjuncts are also helpful in assessing perfusion of bowel-related masses. Fluid-filled dilated small bowel loops in high-grade small-bowel obstruction can also be readily recognised during the transabdominal ultrasound examination.

Image analysis

The normal intestine has a single-wall thickness of 4 mm or less. The normal gut wall has a reproducible pattern of alternating layers appearing as brighter and darker layers on ultrasound, referred to as mural stratification or the 'gut signature'. These layers correspond to the different histological layers of the bowel wall.

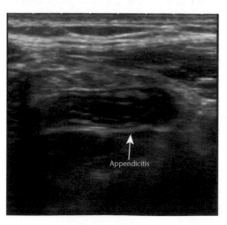

Appendicitis

Figure 5.9 The appendix can be positively identified by following it to its blind end; a non-compressible, thick-walled tubular structure arising from the caecal pole and with a blind end is diagnostic of acute appendicitis.

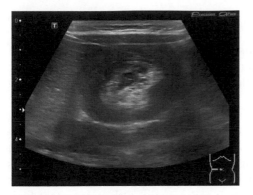

Figure 5.10 A transverse axial image from the right flank shows the typical 'bowel-within-bowel' appearance in intussusception.

Gut-related diseases often result in an abnormally thickened wall that creates recognisable patterns of disease. The possible causes are determined on ultrasound by the location, extent and degree of thickening, along with evaluation of whether the wall thickening is concentric or eccentric and whether there is preservation or disruption of the mural stratification.[6,7]

An abnormally thickened wall is a sign of appendicitis (**Figure 5.9**). Sometimes the bowel will fold into itself, causing intussusception (**Figure 5.10**). This can be seen on ultrasound as a 'target sign' in transverse section, with a thick hyperechoic outer wall. **Figures 5.11** and **5.12** demonstrate a long segment of inflamed oedematous small bowel. The images show symmetrical thickening with preservation of mural stratification in longitudinal and transverse sections, respectively. These appearances are suggestive of inflammatory or ischaemic

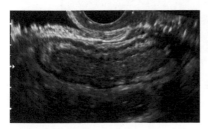

Figure 5.11 Longitudinal section of bowel showing inflammatory change due to Crohn's disease.

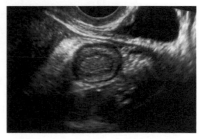

Figure 5.12 Transverse section of bowel showing inflammatory change due to Crohn's disease.

thickening. In this case, the thickening was inflammatory and due to Crohn's disease.

Conversely, neoplastic disease usually affects a short segment of bowel and the thickening can be asymmetrical, irregular and eccentric or annular. Disruption of the gut-wall layers suggests an underlying neoplastic process; in **Figure 5.13** this is a colonic carcinoma. These are general guidelines rather than absolute rules; for example, thickening due to sigmoid diverticulitis can mimic the neoplastic process.

Assessment of extramural changes, particularly the peri-enteric fat, may indicate underlying bowel pathology. Inflamed oedematous fat is characteristically hyperechoic and produces a mass effect. This makes the abnormal bowel more conspicuous. Other important findings include enlarged mesenteric lymph nodes, fluid collections and increased flow in the vasa recta.

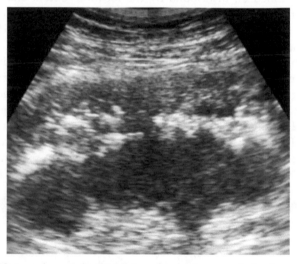

Figure 5.13 Irregular annular thickening of a short segment of colon with loss of stratification.

ENDOSCOPIC ULTRASOUND (EUS)

Transcutaneous sonography is a well-established imaging modality but is limited by poor visualisation of deep structures, especially in the larger patient, due to the inverse relationship between the quality of the image produced and the depth of penetration of the sound waves. In addition, the image is impaired by intervening bowel and gas, bone or other structures.

Technology has evolved, enabling the incorporation of small ultrasound transducers into endoscopes, allowing access to deep structures adjacent to the upper and lower GI tract, as well as imaging of the gut wall itself. Because only a small depth of penetration is required, high-frequency ultrasound can provide improved image resolution. The great advantage of EUS over traditional (optical) endoscopy is the ability to image beyond the surface of the gut, enabling assessment of tumour depth and invasiveness.

Indications

Endoscopic sonography can provide detailed imaging of mediastinal masses, retroperitoneal lymphadenopathy and the pancreas. Tiny stones in the gallbladder, which may be missed on conventional ultrasound, can be identified as well as small stones within the distal bile duct, an area often obscured by bowel gas transabdominally.

High-resolution imaging of the individual layers of the intestinal wall is possible, allowing depth of any tumours to be assessed in the parts of the GI tract accessible at endoscopy (oesophagus, stomach, duodenum, rectum and anus). This improves tumour staging and guides treatment.

It is possible to perform fine-needle aspiration cytology (FNAC) of small or previously inaccessible structures by passing the thin needle under ultrasound guidance through the gut wall and into adjacent structures to diagnose tumours or other pathology. As well as diagnosis by imaging with or without FNAC, EUS can be used to guide drainage of cysts and abscesses and to perform retroperitoneal nerve blocks for chronic pain.

EUS is also being developed to facilitate the delivery of targeted chemotherapy, whereby drug-eluting microbeads can be delivered more directly to the liver. This may be beneficial even for diffuse hepatic metastases, with fewer systemic side effects.[8]

Patient preparation

- Patients undergoing upper GI endoscopic sonography are starved for 4 hours prior to the procedure, which is performed under light sedation, and takes 15–60 minutes depending on interventions performed.
- Drainage of cysts requires antibiotic prophylaxis.
- Transrectal EUS requires a phosphate enema to clear the rectum and sigmoid colon, and rarely requires sedation.

Imaging procedure

Two basic scanning methods exist. Mechanically rotating or radial transducers produce a 360° image perpendicular to the long axis of the endoscope. Convex phased array scanners produce a sector image (100–120°) parallel to the axis of the scope. Although orientation is more difficult with the latter, FNAC is easier because the needle can be visualised and followed during its whole traverse.[9] Both types of echo-endoscopes have forward-oblique viewing systems enabling an endoscopic view of the gut as well as an ultrasound image. A balloon at the tip of the echo-endoscope is inflated with water to provide a sonic window, producing clearer images. The transducers operate at frequencies of 7.5–12 MHz, compared with 2.5–5 MHz in conventional ultrasound, with marked increases in image resolution. The effective image range is usually up to 5 or 6 cm.[10,11]

Colourflow Doppler helps differentiate vessels and clarifies the anatomy. Imaging is performed via the oesophagus to obtain views of the mediastinum and oesophageal wall via the stomach, to image the liver, spleen, kidneys, adrenal glands, retroperitoneal lymph nodes and masses, body and tail of pancreas and stomach wall itself. Imaging via the duodenum produces detailed images of the head of the pancreas, gallbladder and ducts. Transrectal or transanal EUS allows imaging of polyps, pelvic structures and anal sphincters.

Post-procedure, patients usually rest for 1–2 hours before going home.

Image analysis

Figures 5.14 to **5.16** have been obtained using an annular array, the type of transducer described above. This produces a 360° image that is essentially a cross-section of the anatomy immediately surrounding the transducer, which is located in the central anechoic (black) area of the image.

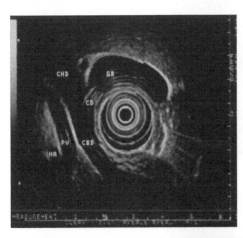

Figure 5.14 (left) Normal biliary tree imaged via the duodenal bulb.
CBD, common bile duct
CD, cystic duct
CHD, common hepatic duct
GB, gallbladder
HA, hepatic artery
PV, portal vein.

Figure 5.15 (right) A stone in the common bile duct (CBD) (green callipers).

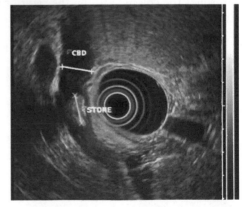

A gallstone in the biliary duct system often causes dilatation, as demonstrated in **Figure 5.15** in the upper left portion of the image. The stone is casting an acoustic shadow, which is the anechoic (darker) area to the left of the image.

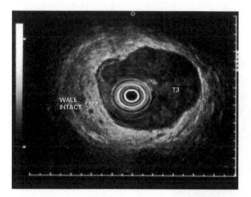

Figure 5.16 Retrograde endoscopic ultrasound of the colon.

The image in **Figure 5.16** has been produced by retrograde EUS of the colon, and shows a cross-section of the colon at the point where a tumour has breached the colonic wall. Note that the colonic wall layers can be seen intact on the left side of the image, and the tumour breaches the colonic wall on the right of the image; this is a T3 or T4 tumour, according to the tumour, node, metastases (TNM) grading system.[12]

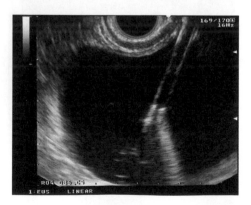

Figure 5.17 Pancreatic pseudocyst drainage.

Figure 5.17 is an image produced by a micro-convex array transducer; note the basic sector shape. This demonstrates how ultrasound can be used to enable visualisation of a needle advanced into the optimum position for the drainage of a pancreatic pseudocyst, for content analysis and symptom relief. The needle is clearly seen within the anechoic area prior to aspiration.

THE NEONATAL GI TRACT

Advances in neonatal care in recent years have increased the survival of more preterm and term-delivered but ill babies. Consequently, there has been a shift from respiratory to GI disorders as a key factor in mortality and morbidity. The small size of newborn babies allows evaluation of the entire depth of the abdomen by ultrasound. It is non-invasive and can be performed at the cot side with no radiation exposure as compared with other means of abdominal imaging, in keeping with the goals of the Image Gently campaign.[13] Sonography also allows a functional assessment of the abdomen that is not possible with standard radiography.[14]

Indications

Neonatal abdominal sonography is used to image both congenital and acquired conditions. Congenital anomalies are usually obstructive in nature, presenting for the first time shortly after birth, for example volvulus, although some antenatally detected conditions may require confirmation and further evaluation postnatally. Acquired disorders usually relate to prematurity and its complications, the most severe one being necrotising enterocolitis (NEC).

Patient preparation

No specific preparation of the patient is required, but newborn babies are very susceptible to cold, and every effort should be made to minimise heat loss during the examination. Warmed bottled gel may pose an infection risk, so a single-use sachet of sterile coupling gel should be pre-warmed to avoid cold stress. Newborns can easily be examined in an open cot or incubator. Good communication with the neonatal team looking after the newborn will help avoid safety hazards and allow more efficient imaging. For example, interventions, which are not life sustaining may be suspended briefly to undertake sonography.

The utmost hand hygiene should always be observed when examining newborns. Before and after examining the newborn, the machine, probe and cable should be cleaned in accordance with evidence-based protocols.

Imaging procedure

When first examining a newborn, all of the intra-abdominal organs should be visualised, recorded and documented using standard views. Using coupling gel, a linear array probe with a transducer frequency of at least 7.5 MHz is placed gently on the upper abdomen and moved in a systematic manner to image the abdominal contents (**Figure 5.18**). Additional views for particular structures or diagnostic questions, for example pyloric stenosis, may be necessary. Other views are possible, as appropriate to the initial request or clinical question, the age of the patient, pathological findings and judgement of the sonographer. Bowel gas compromises sonographic imaging, but much of it may be displaced by applying gently graded compression using the probe.[15] Pathologies must be imaged in two planes, and documented in the report.

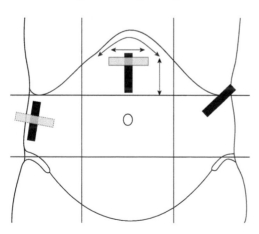

Figure 5.18 Diagram of the abdomen with the probe positions represented as grey and black rectangles, and the movements (arrows) used to obtain the different views.

Image analysis

Figure 5.19 shows normal neonatal gut, whereas **Figure 5.20** shows irregularly shaped, markedly thickened, poorly demarcated bowel wall, which has a heterogeneous echotexture with brighter spots. These findings are suggestive of an inflammatory bowel condition such as NEC.

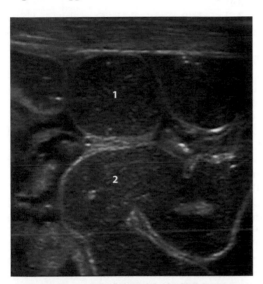

Figure 5.19 Normal, slightly dilated loops of bowel seen in transverse (1) and longitudinal (2) sections filled with stool. Note the regular, moderately thin and well-demarcated bowel wall with homogeneous echotexture.

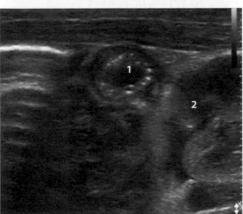

Figure 5.20 Small bowel loops in transverse (1) and longitudinal (2) sections. There is again some slight dilatation but note the echoes in the thickened walls giving a very different appearance from **Figure 5.19**.

REFERENCES

1. Katz P, Hartl DM, Guerre A. Clinical ultrasound of the salivary glands. *Otolaryngologic Clinics of North America* 2009;**42**(6):973–1000. doi: 10.1016/j.otc.2009.08.009.

2. Bialek EJ, Jakubowski W, Zajkowski P, Szopinski K, Osmolski A. US of the major salivary glands: Anatomy and spatial relationships, pathologic conditions and pitfalls. *Radiographics* 2006;**26**(3):745–763. doi: 10.1148/rg.263055024.

3. Schapher M, Goncalves M, Mantsopoulos K, Iro H, Koch M. Transoral ultrasound: A helpful and easy diagnostic method in obstructive salivary gland diseases. *European Radiology* 2019;**29**(7):3635–3637. doi: 10.1007/s00330-019-06201-z.

4. Stefanac SJ, Nesbit SP. *Diagnosis and treatment planning in dentistry*, 3rd edn. St. Louis, MO: Elsevier, 2016.

5. Białek EJ, Jakubowski W. Mistakes in ultrasound examination of salivary glands. *Journal of Ultrasonography* 2016;**16**(65):191–203. doi: 10.15557/JoU.2016.0020.

6. Kuzmich S, Howlett DC, Andi A, Shah D, Kuzmich T. Transabdominal sonography in assessment of the bowel in adults. *American Journal of Roentgenology* 2009;**192**(1):197–212. doi: 10.2214/AJR.07.3555.

7. Maturen KE, Wasnik AP, Kamaya A, Dillman JR, Kaza RK, Pandya A, et al. Ultrasound imaging of bowel pathology: Technique and keys to diagnosis in the acute abdomen. *American Journal of Roentgenology* 2011;**197**(6):1067–1075. doi: 10.2214/AJR.11.6594.

8. Luthra AK, Evans JA. Review of current and evolving clinical indications for endoscopic ultrasound. *World Journal of Gastrointestinal Endoscopy* 2016;**8**(3):157–164. doi: 10.4253/wjge.v8.i3.157.

9. Mallery S. Endoscopic instrumentation. In: Shami VM, Kahaleh M, (eds), *Endoscopic ultrasound*. New York: Springer, 2010:3–32.

10. Lingenfelser T, Guenther E, Piacentino F. 7090 7.5 MHz catheter probe ultrasonography of the upper gastrointestinal tract: A comparison with standard endoscopic ultrasonography. *Gastrointestinal Endoscopy* 2000;**51**(4):AB264. doi: 10.1016/S0016-5107(00)14761-3.

11. Mekky MA, Abbas WA. Endoscopic ultrasound in gastroenterology: From diagnosis to therapeutic implications. *World Journal of Gastroenterology* 2014;**20**(24):7801–7807. doi: 10.3748/wjg.v20.i24.7801.

12. Bowel Cancer UK. *Staging sand grading*. 2019. Available at: https://www.bowelcanceruk.org.uk/about-bowel-cancer/diagnosis/staging-and-grading.

13. Goske MJ, Applegate KE, Boylan J, Butler PF, Callahan MJ, Coley BD, et al. The Image Gently campaign: Working together to change practice. *American Journal of Roentgenology* 2008;**190**(2):273–274. doi: 10.2214/AJR.07.3526.

14. Willis CE, Slovis TL. The ALARA concept in pediatric CR and DR: Dose reduction in pediatric radiographic exams – a white paper conference executive summary. *Pediatric Radiology* 2004;**34**(Suppl 3):S162–S164. doi: 10.1007/s00247-004-1264-y.

15. Gale HI, Gee MS, Westra SJ, Nimkin K. Abdominal ultrasonography of the pediatric gastrointestinal tract. *World Journal of Radiology* 2016;**8**(7):656–667. doi: 10.4329/wjr.v8.i7.656.

Further reading

Penman I, Norton S, Harris K. *Staging of oesophago-gastric carcinoma by endoscopic ultrasonography: Guidance and minimum standards.* London: UK Endoscopic Ultrasound Users Group, 2004:1–21.

Sanders R, Hall-Terracciano B. *Clinical sonography,* 5th edn. London: Lippincott, Williams & Wilkins, 2015.

CHAPTER 6

ENDOCRINE SYSTEM – THYROID AND ADRENAL GLANDS

The thyroid gland   128
The adrenal glands   135
References   139

THE THYROID GLAND

The thyroid gland is a superficial, soft-tissue structure located in the neck, anterior to the trachea. It is part of the endocrine system. Due to its superficial location and soft-tissue nature, it is accessible to examination by high-frequency ultrasound.

As with any ultrasound examination, a good knowledge of relevant anatomy is essential. The anatomy of the thyroid gland itself is not complex, although an understanding of thyroid embryology will aid understanding of anatomical variants and pathology. The anatomy of the surrounding structures of the head and neck should also be understood, as the whole neck should be assessed thoroughly.

Indications

The most common indications for thyroid ultrasound are:

- palpable neck mass;
- elevated serum calcium levels;
- possible parathyroid mass;
- incidental focal thyroid lesions on CT or MR scans.

Other uses are to triage patients into those requiring fine-needle aspiration (FNA) of focal thyroid lesions and those who require no diagnostic intervention. There is also a role for ultrasound after thyroid surgery in detecting postoperative complications, recurrence of thyroid nodules or in the case of thyroidectomy for Graves' disease, recurrence of thyroid tissue.

Patient preparation

The patient is required to remove clothing and jewellery from around the neck region. Long hair should also be moved away from the area of interest. An examination gown should be provided in some cases, bearing in mind that enlarged thyroid glands often demonstrate retrosternal extension and thyroid ultrasound will often lead to examination of other structures within the neck, and should always include regional lymph nodes.

Imaging procedure

The patient lies supine on the examination couch with a pillow underneath the shoulders. Some degree of neck extension is required for a good thyroid examination, but the patient should not be uncomfortable. If this position is difficult to attain, for example in elderly people or those with cervical arthritis, the head of the ultrasound couch can be raised to about 45°, which may facilitate patient comfort while still allowing for some neck extension. The neck should be assessed in transverse and longitudinal sections.

A high-frequency linear array transducer is selected, usually 10–12 MHz. Scanning should begin in the lower part of the anterior neck, just below the cricoid cartilage, with the probe in a transverse orientation, to see the thyroid isthmus (**Figure 6.1**). Starting with the right lobe of the thyroid, the probe is moved slightly lateral from the starting position and angled towards the midline of the neck just enough to maintain contact between the neck and the probe surface. This demonstrates the right lobe of the thyroid and its surrounding structures in transverse section. Moving the probe cranially and caudally in this plane ensures visualisation of both upper and lower poles of the thyroid in transverse section. Turning the probe 90° enables a longitudinal image of the right lobe of the thyroid to be obtained. Slight rocking of the probe in this plane ensures imaging of the whole thyroid in longitudinal section. This procedure is repeated for the left lobe (**Figure 6.2**).

Although the parathyroid glands may in theory be identified in this region, in practice they are often difficult to see even with the use of

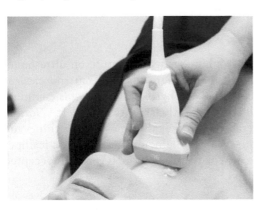

Figure 6.1 Positioning of probe for a transverse section.

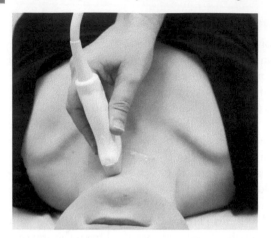

Figure 6.2 Positioning of probe for a longitudinal section.

high-frequency transducers, unless they are enlarged, for instance by an adenoma.

The addition of colourflow Doppler to the B mode technique is useful to delineate blood vessels and assess overall blood flow within the thyroid gland. This may contribute to the decision-making process of whether to refer a patient with focal lesions or to extend the examination to include an FNA.

Images should be recorded of the thyroid isthmus in transverse section, both lobes of the thyroid in transverse and longitudinal section and any additional pathology such as enlarged lymph nodes. The anteroposterior (AP) diameters of both thyroid lobes and any identified focal lesions should be measured.

Image analysis

The normal thyroid gland has a homogeneous texture on ultrasound, its echogenicity being higher than the overlying strap muscles, as demonstrated in **Figures 6.3** and **6.4**. Thyroid asymmetry is common, with the right lobe generally being slightly larger than the left.[1] Normal thyroid size varies considerably and depends, among other things, on patient gender and physique. An AP diameter measurement (calliper placement shown in **Figure 6.5**) of 18 mm or more is generally accepted to represent an enlarged gland.[2,3]

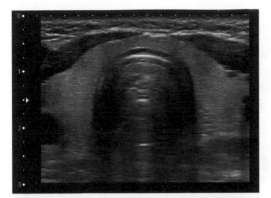

Figure 6.3 Transverse section through a normal thyroid, demonstrating the normal homogeneous thyroid texture and echogenicity relative to the anterior strap muscles, and the relationship of surrounding structures.

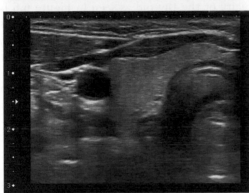

Figure 6.4 Transverse section through the thyroid, showing a normal right lobe and the adjacent anechoic, rounded, common carotid artery.

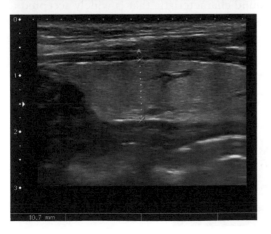

Figure 6.5 Longitudinal section of the right thyroid lobe with AP measurement.

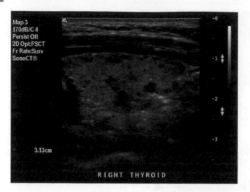

Figure 6.6 Thyroid demonstrating diffuse changes in echogenicity.

Diffuse altered echogenicity of the thyroid as seen in **Figure 6.6** is frequently encountered, particularly in autoimmune diseases such as Graves' disease and Hashimoto's thyroiditis. In these clinical scenarios, the thyroid can be enlarged, normal in size or atrophic, and hyper- or hypovascular, depending on disease stage. Subacute (viral) thyroiditis often presents with a focal area of altered echogenicity within the thyroid, but the gland itself usually returns back to normal after 6 months.[1]

Identification of focal lesions is probably the most important role of thyroid ultrasound and the goal of the examination is to exclude a thyroid malignancy. This can be particularly challenging in multinodular goitres, when the thyroid is enlarged by multiple nodules (**Figure 6.7**). One ultrasound characteristic that is widely accepted to denote a benign nodule is that of the 'spongiform appearance' as seen in **Figure 6.8**.[4] A completely hyperechoic nodule is also likely to be benign.[5]

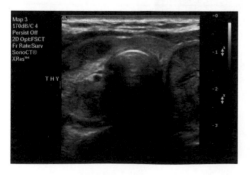

Figure 6.7 Multinodular goitre; enlargement of both lobes of the thyroid, with multiple nodules.

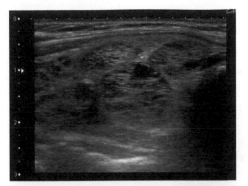

Figure 6.8 Nodule with a 'spongiform pattern', likely to be benign.

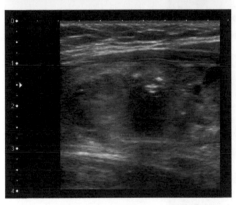

Figure 6.9 A nodule of indeterminate appearance; in this instance fine-needle aspiration would follow.

It is often not possible to exclude a malignancy with imaging alone and suspicious lesions are referred for FNA under ultrasound guidance. An example of such a nodule of indeterminate appearance is shown in **Figure 6.9**. Ultrasound findings increasing suspicion of malignancy are: a hypoechoic lesion, the presence of microcalcification (not to be confused with the echogenic foci demonstrating comet-tail artefacts in benign colloid nodules as seen in **Figure 6.10**), central rather than peripheral vascularity, a 'taller than wide' nodule, irregular margins, incomplete halo and documented enlargement.[6] The Ultrasound (U) Classification system can be used to assist in deciding whether to continue to FNA, depending on lesion characteristics.[4] This system suggests normal (U1), benign (U2), indeterminate (U3), suspicious (U4) and malignant (U5) likelihood based on ultrasound appearances.

Abnormal enlarged lymph nodes (**Figure 6.11**), usually taller than they are wide, also assist in determining likelihood of malignancy.

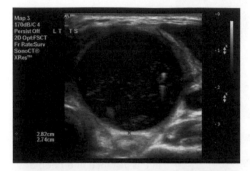

Figure 6.10 A benign (U2) colloid nodule in the left lobe of thyroid. A comet-tail artefact can be seen on the right side of the image, within the anechoic, smooth-walled cystic lesion.

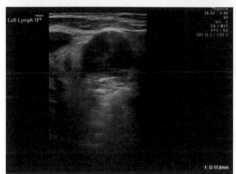

Figure 6.11 An enlarged left-sided lymph node in the neck.

Extended field of view ultrasound or trapezoidal feature on a linear array transducer can be useful to provide a wider field of view. This enables comparison of the appearances of both lobes of thyroid and assessment of the extent of a lesion.

THE ADRENAL GLANDS

The adrenal glands are situated medial to the upper poles of the kidneys. Because of their position high in the abdomen and adjacent to the spine, they can easily be obscured by the ribs, bowel gas, the transverse processes of the vertebrae and perinephric fat. Therefore, unless they are enlarged, the adrenal glands can be challenging to image with ultrasound, particularly the left adrenal gland.[7] If seen, they are often triangular, with a hypoechoic centre and hyperechoic outline.

Indications

Because of the above difficulties, ultrasound is not generally indicated for investigations of the adrenal glands in the adult, although they may be seen occasionally during EUS (endoscopic ultrasound), and are commonly seen in young infants. Most findings are therefore incidental during examination of the kidneys or other abdominal viscera, and it is important to include the adrenal region, as most adrenal pathology is asymptomatic.

Patient preparation

No special preparation is needed to scan the adrenal glands, although being nil by mouth for a few hours beforehand may limit the amount of bowel content and so assist visualisation. As with other abdominal ultrasound examinations, the clothing should be removed from the area, with a gown provided if necessary for the patient's privacy and dignity.

Imaging procedure

Using a curvilinear array transducer of 2.5–5 MHz, the adrenal glands are examined with the patient either turned 45° on to the side (posterior oblique position) or lying completely on the side (lateral decubitus position) as in **Figures 6.12** and **6.13**. The upper abdominal viscera may be used as acoustic windows to aid visualization, the liver for the right and the spleen for the left, with a subcostal approach as shown in **Figures 6.12** and **6.13**.

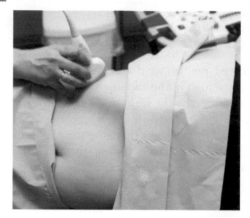

Figure 6.12 (left) Patient in the left lateral decubitus position for the right adrenal gland.

Figure 6.13 (right) Patient in the right lateral decubitus position for the left adrenal gland.

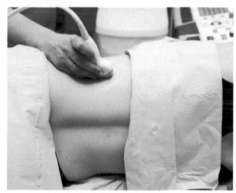

If there is gas obscuring the adrenal glands an intercostal approach may help, the probe being positioned at the ninth and tenth intercostal space in the midaxillary line on the raised side. Alternatively, the patient may lie supine and be scanned in the midaxillary line with the probe directed horizontally.

The adrenal glands should be found superior to the kidney, between the diaphragm and the liver or spleen. A series of transverse images is produced from the renal hilum inferiorly to a level several centimetres superior to the kidney to completely cover the adrenal area, and the probe rotated through 90° to ensure complete coverage in two orthogonal planes.[8]

Image analysis

The liver makes a good acoustic window for the right adrenal gland and right kidney, as shown in **Figure 6.14**, which is a section obtained from the position shown in **Figure 6.12**. This is a coronal (longitudinal) section and shows a normal adrenal gland (rounded structure beyond the upper pole of the kidney).

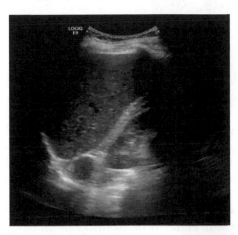

Figure 6.14 (left) A coronal section of the liver, right adrenal gland and kidney.

Figure 6.15 (right). A similar section, showing a benign adenoma of the right adrenal gland, measuring 2.5 cm.

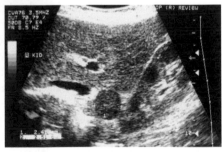

An adrenal adenoma is a common finding, increasingly so with age, and appears as a homogeneous and hypoechoic solid lesion with well-defined borders and hypovascularisation. This is seen in **Figure 6.15**, a longitudinal section obtained from a slightly more anterior aspect than that in **Figure 6.14**. An adenoma may appear very similar to the normal adrenal gland, and power Doppler (not shown here) should be applied to any suspicious mass seen to ascertain vascularisation.

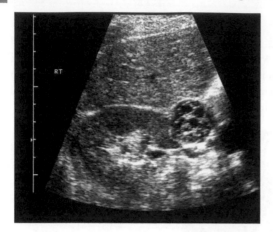

Figure 6.16 A transverse section showing the liver, the right kidney and a phaeochromocytoma of the right adrenal gland (rounded heterogeneous mass medial to the kidney).

Ultrasound can easily differentiate between cystic and solid adrenal lesions; simple cysts are uncommon and usually benign. The sensitivity and specificity of ultrasound in the differentiation of solid adrenal lesions has improved in recent years, and the characteristics are described as follows:[9]

- Phaeochromocytomas are well encapsulated and mostly of mixed echotexture, as demonstrated in **Figure 6.16**. Normal adrenal tissue cannot itself be identified on this image. Pheochromocytomas typically have increased vascularity apparent on power Doppler.
- A myelolipoma appears hyperechoic because of its fat content, with smooth margins and low vascularity.
- An adrenocortical carcinoma generally appears as a large heterogeneous, solid mass at the time of diagnosis, with hypervascularisation.
- An adrenal metastasis (**Figure 6.17**), the commonest malignant finding, usually has an irregular outline and echotexture, with increased vascularisation, although appearances may vary widely.

Unidentified adrenal masses can be sampled by ultrasound-guided FNA to obtain a sample for histological diagnosis in the case of adrenal masses.

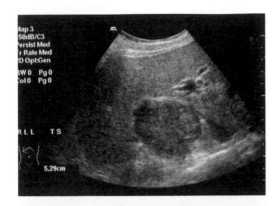

Figure 6.17 A metastatic mass in the adrenal gland.

REFERENCES

1. Ahuja A, Evans R. *Practical Head and Neck Ultrasound.* Cambridge: Cambridge University Press, 2000.
2. Lupo M. *Thyroid Cancer/Nodules and Hyperthyroidism Expert Forum,* 2005. www.Medhelp.org/posts/Thyroid-Cancer-Nodules-Hyperthyroidism/Normal-Thyroid-Size/show/263195.
3. Unattributed at the University of Virginia. *Thyroid Ultrasound.* 2013. https://www.med-ed.virginia.edu/courses/rad/Thyroid_Ultrasound/01intro/intro-01-02.html.
4. Perros P, Colley S, Boelaert K, et al. British Thyroid Association Guidelines for the Management of Thyroid Cancer. *Clinical Endocrinology* 2014; **81**(S1);1–122.
5. Bonavita J, Mayo J, Babb J, et al. Pattern recognition of benign nodules at ultrasound of the thyroid: Which nodules can be left alone? *American Journal of Radiology* 2009;**193**:207-213.
6. Blum M. *Ultrasonography of the Thyroid on Thyroid Disease Manager,* 2010. www.thyroidmanager.org/chapter/ultrasonography-of-the-thyroid.
7. Słapa RZ, Jakubowski WS, Dobruch-Sobczak K, Kasperlik-Załuska AA. Standards of ultrasound imaging of the adrenal glands. *Journal of Ultrasonography* 2015;**15**(63):377–387. doi: 10.15557/JoU.2015.0035.
8. Nürnberg D, Szebeni A, Zát'ura F. *Ultrasound of the adrenal glands; EFSUMB – European Course Book,* 2011. www.kosmos-design.co.uk/EFSUMB-ECB/ecb-ch013-adrenal.pdf.

References

9. Fan J, Tang J, Fang J, et al. Ultrasound imaging in the diagnosis of benign and suspicious adrenal lesions. *Medical Science Monitor* 2014;**20**: 2132–2141. doi: 10.12659/MSM.890800.

CHAPTER 7

THE FEMALE REPRODUCTIVE SYSTEM

Gynaecological ultrasound   142
Hysterosalpingo-contrast sonography (HyCoSy)   152
Assisted reproduction   157
References   161

GYNAECOLOGICAL ULTRASOUND

Ultrasound is the most commonly used method of imaging the female pelvis, because there is no radiation risk to the reproductive organs or to a possible fetus. Images may be obtained transabdominally using a 3.5–5 MHz curvilinear probe, although transvaginal ultrasound is the method of choice for accurate diagnostic imaging for gynaecological purposes. This method, sometimes also known as endovaginal or endocavity sonography, uses a high-frequency (7.5 MHz) dedicated transvaginal probe (**Figure 7.1**). The transvaginal approach gives improved image resolution due to the closer proximity of the transducer to the pelvic organs, as the tip is inserted into the vagina to about 5–8 cm. Occasionally both techniques may be employed to ensure a comprehensive examination.

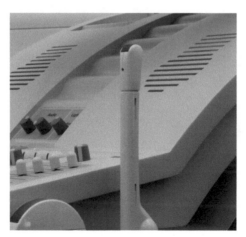

Figure 7.1 Transvaginal probe.

Indications

Women may be referred for investigation of:
- palpable or suspected pelvic mass or swelling;
- pelvic pain;

- menstrual disturbances;
- location of intrauterine contraceptive devices;
- suspicion of retained products of conception;
- postmenopausal bleeding;
- strong family history of ovarian carcinoma;
- abnormal tests, for instance cancer antigen 125 (CA125), or raised levels of human chorionic gonadotrophin (hCG) in the absence of pregnancy.

Patient preparation

For transabdominal ultrasound of the pelvis, a full bladder is required. This elevates the uterus, displaces bowel gas, provides an acoustic window to allow visualisation of pelvic structures and provides an anatomical reference point.

Conversely, an empty bladder facilitates access to the uterus and is more comfortable for a transvaginal examination, so the patient is asked to empty her bladder immediately prior to the examination. Strict clean technique must be followed when using the transvaginal probe. Gloves must be worn by the sonographer, and it is important to check with the patient if she has a sensitivity or allergy to latex, so that non-latex gloves and probe covers are used for the examination.

As always, a full explanation of the procedure and techniques must be given to the patient and her consent obtained. This is of particular importance in transvaginal scanning, as patients may not be aware of the intimate nature of the examination. It is also the right of the patient and the sonographer to have a chaperone present for the examination.

A full history should be taken, including the menstrual status, as the appearance of the endometrium and ovaries will vary throughout the menstrual cycle in women of reproductive age, as represented in **Figure 7.2**. It is also important to note any relevant surgery and to ask about contraceptive use, including hormonal treatments, contraceptive devices and drug therapy, as certain pharmaceuticals can affect the ultrasound appearances of the endometrium (e.g. tamoxifen) and ovaries (e.g. clomiphene).

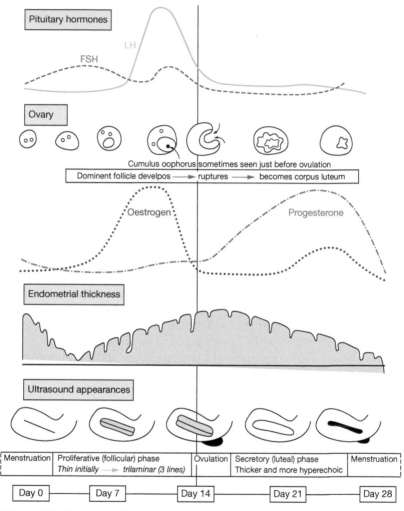

Figure 7.2 Changes in ultrasound appearances of the endometrium and ovaries in relation to the menstrual cycle and hormonal fluctuations. FSH, follicle-stimulating hormone; LH, luteinising hormone.

Imaging procedure

Transabdominal: with the patient supine on the examination couch and coupling gel applied, longitudinal images are obtained by holding the probe in the midline sagittal plane just superior to the symphysis pubis. Parasagittal sections are then obtained by moving the probe in a continuous scanning action to each side of the lower abdomen and pelvis.

The probe is rotated through 90° and transverse images of the lower abdomen are achieved, starting at the symphysis pubis and moving the probe cranially with a continuous scanning action.

Once the regions of interest have been identified, additional oblique scan sections are required to complete the examination.

Transvaginal: because of the nature of the procedure, stringent steps must be taken to prevent cross-contamination. Before insertion into the vagina, ultrasound gel is applied to the probe, which is then inserted into a sterile cover. Sterile gel is then applied to the tip of the covered probe. To prevent contamination, the transducer must be cleaned after every examination in accordance with the manufacturer's instructions.

The patient lies supine on the examination couch with her feet supported and the lower limbs in a position to facilitate a transvaginal examination. The probe is introduced gently into the vagina and carefully manoeuvred to visualise the anatomical structures in sagittal section. Keeping the thumb on the anterior aspect of the probe enables the alignment to be judged when rotating the probe during the examination. The probe is angled anteriorly and posteriorly, and rotated to visualise the long axis of the uterus for the endometrium to be assessed and measured. The probe is then rotated anticlockwise through 90° to examine the uterus in its short axis. From this position, the probe is angled towards the adnexae and the ovaries identified, measured and assessed.

In transvaginal ultrasound, the probe orientation for optimal views may be incompatible with alignment with anatomical planes, and this may result in some confusion when viewing images. Therefore, it is particularly important that images are annotated correctly regarding orientation.

During gynaecological sonography using either technique, the size, shape, outline and echotexture of the pelvic organs are examined and measurements taken. Subtle changes in echotexture of the uterine parenchyma can indicate pathology such as fibroids or adenomyosis. The adnexae are assessed for evidence of fluid collections or hydrosalpinx. The operator records images of any abnormality, with measurements as appropriate. Colourflow and power Doppler can be used to assess vascularity and aid in the diagnosis of suspected masses, as in other areas of the body.

Image analysis

A midline transvaginal scan demonstrating the long axis (sagittal section) of the uterus and endometrium is important to demonstrate the uterine echotexture (**Figure 7.3**). Measurements of the uterine length and anteroposterior (AP) diameter are taken. The endometrium is assessed and measured at its maximum AP thickness. **Figure 7.3** is an anteverted uterus and the appearances in this image are normal. The thin endometrium is normal for the early proliferative stage of the menstrual cycle (days 1–6). The hypoechoic area in the myometrium at the fundus is artefactual – this exemplifies why images are best viewed in real time and interpreted by the operator.

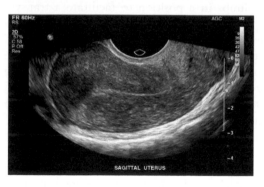

Figure 7.3 Transvaginal scan of an anteverted uterus.

The retroverted uterus in **Figure 7.4** has the fundus of the uterus as the curvature to the right of the image, whereas in **Figures 7.3** and **7.5** this is shown to the left of the image. In a retroverted uterus, the anterior uterine wall is demonstrated on the posterior aspect of the image. The endometrium in **Figure 7.4** is thickened, with some fluid areas present within it. The measurement is shown as 1.74 cm (17.4 mm); it should be no more than 16 mm in women of reproductive age at any stage of their cycle,[1] so this demonstrates endometrial hyperplasia, which would require further investigation, probably by endometrial biopsy to obtain a sample for histology.[2] In postmenopausal women, the normal maximum endometrial thickness is regarded as up to 5 mm.[3]

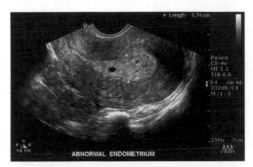

Figure 7.4 Transvaginal scan of a retroverted uterus.

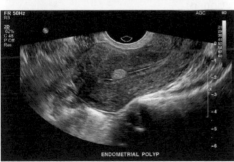

Figure 7.5 Transvaginal scan demonstrating an endometrial polyp

The anteverted uterus in **Figure 7.5** demonstrates a trilaminar appearance of the endometrium (late proliferative stage, days 7–14), interrupted by a brighter (hyperechoic) oval area in the centre of the image. This has the appearance of an endometrial polyp.

Fibroids are commonly seen in women as hypoechoic focal lesions within the myometrium. Fibroids can cause menorrhagia (heavy menstrual bleeding) and dysmenorrhoea (painful periods). They are more frequent in African–Caribbean women and often seen at a younger age. **Figure 7.6** shows an intramural fibroid as a typical well-circumscribed, hypoechoic, rounded lesion measuring 28.3 mm. This is situated within the posterior myometrium and is causing slight anterior deviation of the endometrium. It is important to define the location of the fibroid within the report, as this can influence management.

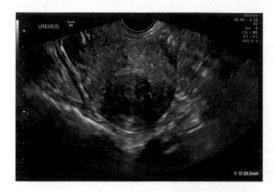

Figure 7.6 Transvaginal image of a uterus containing a fibroid.

Fibroids are defined by location as:

- **intramural** – within the myometrium, as in **Figure 7.6**;
- **submucosal** – growing into the endometrial cavity;
- **subserosal** – protruding from the myometrium and extending beyond the uterine wall;
- **pedunculated** – on a stalk, often outside the uterus. Care must be taken not to mistake these for an ovarian lesion;
- **intracavity** – within the endometrial cavity. These are often pedunculated, but fully within the endometrial cavity.

The introduction of sterile saline is sometimes helpful to delineate structures within the uterine cavity, for example to outline a polyp and distinguish it from an endometrial fibroid or other lesion. Polyps are more likely to be hyperechoic lesions, and sometimes blood flow can be seen in a 'feeder vessel' when applying colourflow Doppler, whereas fibroids are often heterogeneous or hypoechoic.

Fibroids are usually clearly defined focal lesions and should be differentiated from adenomyosis, as the management will be different. Adenomyosis is often mistaken for 'early fibroid change', but this is incorrect. **Figure 7.7** shows thickening of the anterior myometrium, with a generalised heterogeneous echotexture, small cystic areas and vertical linear streaks. When colourflow Doppler is applied, the area shows a generalised hypervascular appearance, as in **Figure 7.8**, whereas a fibroid usually demonstrates peripheral vascularity.

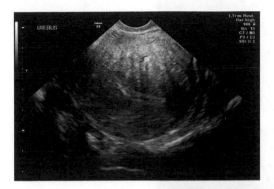

Figure 7.7 (left)
Transvaginal scan of a uterus showing adenomyosis.

Figure 7.8 (right)
Transvaginal scan of a uterus showng the colour Doppler appearances of adenomyosis (same patient as **Figure 7.7**).

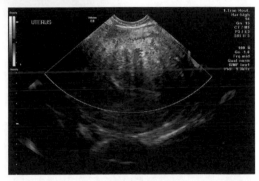

Ultrasound is frequently used to locate intrauterine contraceptive devices when the strings are not located on clinical examination. **Figure 7.9** shows a normal anteverted uterus and endometrium. Within the endometrial cavity are three hyperechoic areas with posterior acoustic shadowing, representing a Mirena intrauterine system (IUS) in the correct position.

Figure 7.10 is a transabdominal scan in a woman of reproductive age. The full bladder is visible as the anterior fluid area and a normal ovary can be seen immediately below it. Around the periphery, the dark areas are developing follicles, one of which will continue to release an ovum.

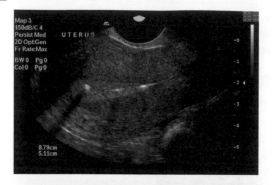

Figure 7.9 Transvaginal scan of a uterus showing a Mirena intrauterine system in situ.

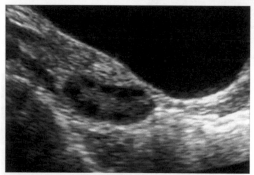

Figure 7.10 Transabdominal scan of an ovary.

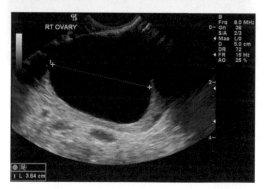

Figure 7.11 A simple ovarian cyst.

A simple ovarian cyst of 3.6 cm is shown in **Figure 7.11**. This is a common appearance in women of reproductive age and is most likely a large follicle that has continued to grow after an egg has been released, and would not in itself warrant follow-up.[4] However, any ovarian mass larger than 5 cm carries a risk of torsion of the ovary,[5] so even a simple cyst over 5 cm would require a follow-up examination.[4]

In **Figure 7.12**, the ovarian tissue is compressed to the periphery of the ovary by an expanded fluid area within an ovarian cyst measuring almost 11 cm in its greatest diameter. There are many possible reasons (differential diagnoses) for this and, although most adnexal masses are ovarian in origin, diagnostic errors can result when this is assumed, rather than proved by the sonographic findings.[5] Therefore, a careful examination of the adnexae is in order whether or not any pathology is seen. In this particular case, there had been a haemorrhage into the cyst.

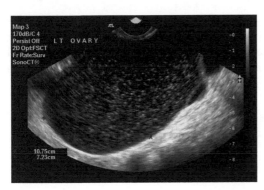

Figure 7.12 Transvaginal scan of an ovarian cyst with internal echoes, suggestive of a haemorrhagic cyst.

Ovarian cysts can be categorised using the 'Assessment of Different NEoplasias in the adneXa (ADNEX)' model, and standardised terminology should be used to report ovarian tumours.[6] **Figure 7.13** demonstrates a 27 cm smooth, multilocular mass with solid tissue present and low-level hyperechoic internal echoes, moderate vascularity, with no ascites. This probably represents a borderline mucinous ovarian tumour. This would need to be confirmed by histology.

Three-dimensional (3D) reconstructions are particularly useful for the pelvic organs,[7] and an example is shown in this chapter in the section on 'Assisted reproduction', where it is often employed for uterine anomalies.

Attention should be given to privacy and dignity at all times. After the procedure, the patient should be provided with tissue to remove the gel and given privacy to dress.

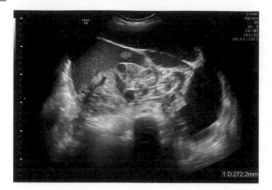

Figure 7.13 Transvaginal scan of a very large ovarian tumour measuring 272mm.

Due to the normal cyclical changes in appearance of the endometrium and ovaries, follow-up ultrasound may be useful to confirm or exclude any equivocal scan findings. This is best done after an interval of around 6 weeks to allow for physiological resolution and to ensure a different phase of the menstrual cycle in women of reproductive age.

HYSTEROSALPINGO-CONTRAST SONOGRAPHY (HyCoSy)

The HyCoSy examination is a dynamic diagnostic examination performed under ultrasound control, similar to the more traditional hysterosalpingography (HSG). HyCoSy obviates the radiation risk of HSG, and research has shown similar pregnancy outcomes.[8] The procedure is undertaken using a special contrast agent such as gel-hydroxyethylcellulose, which is a sugar-based (galactose) solution. It is an effective and well-tolerated procedure.[9]

Indications

HyCoSy is used in many women at the early stage of infertility investigations to demonstrate the appearance of the uterus and ovaries, and to assess the patency of the fallopian tubes. Anomalies such as uterine malformation and damaged or closed tubes have an adverse effect on successful fertilisation and implantation, and can make miscarriage more likely.[10]

Patient preparation

HyCoSy is performed as an outpatient procedure. The woman is asked to take an analgesic shortly before attending for the HyCoSy examination. Ideally, the procedure should be performed early in the menstrual cycle, and the woman should avoid intercourse from the first day of her period until after the examination, as the contrast agent is toxic to the embryo, as well as the physical risks to an early pregnancy. Women who have amenorrhoea or very irregular cycles should have a pregnancy test performed just prior to the examination taking place.

Imaging procedure

The procedure is performed using an aseptic technique. An initial baseline ultrasound scan is performed with the woman in the lithotomy position, the lower limbs supported by leg rests, using a transvaginal probe with a transducer frequency of 7.5 MHz. The uterine size and endometrial thickness are assessed and any structural abnormality outlined. The ovarian sizes are observed and their position and movement relative to the uterus ascertained.

The range of abnormalities that may be seen at this scan can include septate, bicornuate or didelphic uterus, as explained in this chapter in the section on 'Assisted reproduction', and ovarian cysts or masses, polycystic ovaries and hydrosalpinx. HyCoSy is usually contraindicated in cases of hydrosalpinx as well as in cases of known or previous pelvic inflammatory disease, as the contrast agent will not flush freely into the peritoneum, and toxic accumulation must be avoided. Other contraindications at this stage include a stenosed cervix, which would make the examination very difficult if not impossible, and a large pelvic mass, such as a large fibroid or ovarian mass, which could prevent clear visualisation.

The transvaginal probe is then removed and a speculum introduced into the vagina to allow for clear visualisation of the cervix. A balloon catheter is inserted gently through the cervix while checking the woman's comfort level. The balloon is inflated once the catheter has been correctly sited in the uterus. The transvaginal probe is then inserted and the position of the balloon and catheter checked. If a guide was used with the catheter, this is now removed.

The syringe containing the contrast agent should be prepared in accordance with the contrast agent usage instructions. The syringe is now attached to the catheter and the contrast agent introduced into the uterine cavity. The probe is moved to follow the contrast from the uterus along each tube. If they are patent, they fill with the contrast agent and appear as a thin, bright hyperechoic line, which may follow a curved, meandering or reasonably straight path. Careful manipulation of the transvaginal probe allows the flow of the contrast agent to be monitored and recorded.

Flow is checked along to and around each ovary, where the contrast should spill into the peritoneal cavity, being seen as a hyperechoic collection adjacent to the ovary. The flow along the tube is very quick, taking only about 5–15 seconds, unless there is a blockage or if the tube is in spasm. If spasm is a possibility, it is worth reassessing each side after a short interval.

On completion of recording, the probe is removed and the balloon is released and the catheter removed. A vasovagal reaction can occur after the introduction of the contrast agent and after the removal of the catheter, so the woman is advised not to sit up straight away. However, reaction and infection are rare following this procedure.

Image analysis

HyCoSy is a dynamic examination, during which it may take as little as a few seconds for the contrast agent to transit the fallopian tubes, so this is generally viewed in 'real time'. It is difficult to record an examination satisfactorily by still image capture and subsequent viewing, but careful study of the images will reveal the very bright echoes due to the multiple tiny reflectors present in the contrast medium. Recording cine clips can enable review after the procedure.

The catheter and balloon are shown on **Figure 7.14** just as the contrast is introduced into the uterine cavity, as a hyperechoic area within the uterine fundus. In **Figure 7.15** the contrast is visible as a hyperechoic collection around the balloon and in the uterine cavity. After a few seconds of the contrast introduction, **Figures 7.16** and **7.17** demonstrate both fallopian tubes as the contrast medium extends into them. This is seen as thin linear hyperechoic lines. Note the shadowing artefact from the hyperechoic (microbubble) contrast agent in the left cornual area.

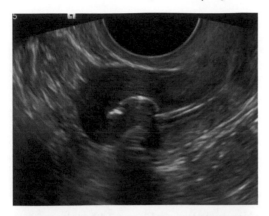

Figure 7.14 Sagittal section of the uterus at early contrast injection.

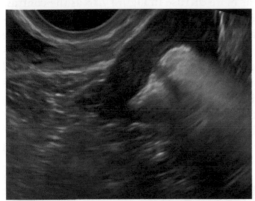

Figure 7.15 Contrast agent filling the uterine cavity; transverse section.

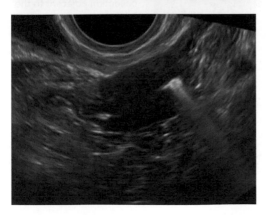

Figure 7.16 Filling in the right tube.

155

Figure 7.17
The left tube fills, with a similar appearance to the right tube, as demonstrated on **Figure 7.16**.

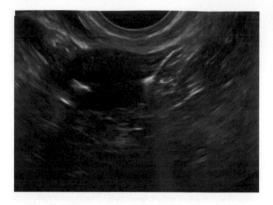

The bright echoes appear more diffuse in **Figure 7.18** as the contrast spreads from the infundibulum of the fallopian tube into the peritoneum. The fact that this happens indicates patency of the fallopian tube on this side. Spill from both sides is the optimum outcome, as one partially or completely blocked fallopian tube may give rise to an increased risk of an ectopic pregnancy. Visualisation of two clear fallopian tubes is a good indication that, if there is a degree of subfertility, this may lie elsewhere. HyCoSy can confirm the normal appearance of the uterus and ovaries along with tubal patency in many women at the early stage of infertility investigations[10] and is thus a milestone on the road to a successful pregnancy.

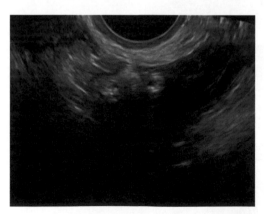

Figure 7.18 A hyperechoic collection adjacent to the left ovary as the contrast spills into the peritoneum.

ASSISTED REPRODUCTION

Ultrasound is the imaging technology of choice for women with fertility issues. It plays a vital role in diagnosis and evaluation of uterine and adnexal pathology: in monitoring the response to gonadotrophins; in egg recovery and embryo transfer; and in early pregnancy assessment. Implantation and pregnancy rates are improved if ultrasound-guided embryo transfer is used in preference to clinical touch methods.[11] Doppler studies of uterine blood flow may provide significant information about endometrial receptivity, failed implantation and early pregnancy loss.[12,13]

Indications

- **Diagnosis and evaluation:** congenital uterine anomalies, fibroids, endometrial polyps, polycystic ovaries, ovarian cysts, endometriosis, antral follicle counts, hydrosalpinx, assessment of tubal patency by HyCoSy and assessment of uterine blood flow.
- **Monitoring:** evaluation of ovarian activity, including follicle tracking, monitoring of the endometrium and assessment of ovarian hyperstimulation syndrome (OHSS).
- **Treatment:** ultrasound plays a vital part in the guidance of oocyte recovery and later embryo transfer.
- **Pregnancy:** detection of fetal heartbeat, dating of pregnancy, diagnosis and management of miscarriage, exclusion of ectopic and heterotopic pregnancy, and determining the chorionicity and amnionicity of multiple gestations.

Patient preparation

A full urinary bladder may be required for the first attendance, although often a series of scans is performed. After an initial transabdominal assessment, the subsequent scans are performed transvaginally, so the woman should attend with an empty bladder for her own comfort.

Imaging procedure

Standard transabdominal and transvaginal techniques for gynaecological sonography are employed, as described in the foregoing section, with a view to evaluating the structure and function of the uterus and ovaries. Scans are often performed daily for monitoring purposes, and this would generally entail an internal scan using a 7.5 MHz transvaginal probe.

Once a pregnancy has been established, routine scans would be performed as for any other pregnancy.

Image analysis

Figures 7.19 and **7.20** are of the same uterus. There is some duplication of anatomy seen in **Figure 7.19**, with two endometrial echoes visible in cross-section. This suggests that there are two uterine cavities, a congenital malformation, which may contribute to reproductive difficulties. It is not possible to determine the exact morphology from this image alone, because two-dimensional (2D) sonography is unable to distinguish reliably bicornuate, septate and didelphic uterus. Uterus didelphys may be confused with a complete uterine septum; similarly, a bicornuate uterus may be confused with an incomplete septum.[14] Correct diagnosis is crucial, as both reproductive prognosis and treatment are anomaly specific. A uterine septum is associated with increased risk of spontaneous miscarriage and removal can improve prognosis, whereas a didelphic or bicornuate uterus is associated with fewer reproductive complications, and unification surgery is technically difficult with variable outcomes.[15]

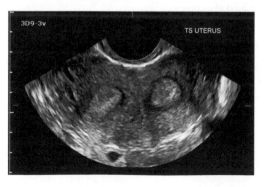

Figure 7.19 A transverse section through the fundus of the uterus, demonstrating two separate endometrial echoes.

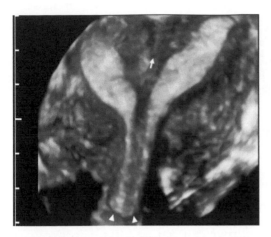

Figure 7.20 The same uterus viewed in a reconstructed coronal plane from three-dimensional sonography, showing the fundal contour (arrow) and double cervix (arrowheads).

Previously, laparoscopy or magnetic resonance imaging (MRI) was necessary for diagnosis, but, with the advent of 3D technology, spatial manipulation of the volume data allows multiplanar views, as shown in **Figure 7.20**, and so congenital uterine anomalies have been easier to classify.[16] In this case, demonstration of the double cervix enabled the correct diagnosis of didelphys bicollis, a complete duplication of uterine horns as well as duplication of the cervix, with no communication between them.

Three-dimensional ultrasound is a less invasive and cheaper modality than MRI and has been shown to have comparable sensitivity and specificity[16,17] and thus plays an important role in evaluating uterine anomalies. If 3D ultrasound is used in combination with saline contrast installation, more accurate localisation of leiomyomas (fibroids) and endometrial polyps is also possible.[18]

Ultrasonic follicle tracking is used in assisted reproduction as a means of monitoring the growth of the ovarian follicles that contain the oocytes. The size and number of the developing follicles can be accurately determined using transvaginal ultrasound, as demonstrated in **Figure 7.21**. Each follicle is identified and displayed in its maximum diameter, and 2D measurements are taken at right angles to each other. The mean of the two measurements is used as the true follicular diameter. The clinician uses the results of sequential scans to optimise the time for the appropriate procedures such as triggering ovulation or performing egg retrieval.

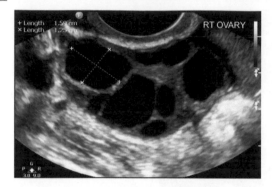

Figure 7.21 Follicle tracking of a gonadotrophin-stimulated ovary, showing calliper placement for follicular measurements.

Pelvic ultrasound may reveal a treatable condition affecting a woman's fertility. For example, an endometrioma, sometimes referred to as a 'chocolate cyst' because of its dark brown colour at surgery, is a cyst arising from growth of ectopic endometrial tissue in the ovary, as in **Figure 7.22**. Treatment options can be surgical or medical, and the decision to treat often depends on the degree and complications of endometrial implants in the pelvis, which can be determined only by laparoscopy. Conservation of fertility is of prime consideration in these women. This is just one of many possible conditions compromising female reproductive capacity that can be diagnosed and managed using ultrasound.

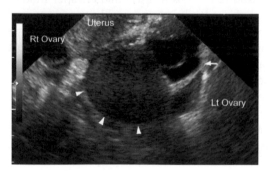

Figure 7.22 Endometrioma (arrowheads) in a gonadotrophin-stimulated left (Lt) ovary. Normal (stimulated) follicles are shown to the right (Rt) of the image by the single arrow.

All images in this section on 'Assisted reproduction' are reproduced with kind permission from CARE Fertility, Manchester.

REFERENCES

1. Tsuda H, Ito YM, Todo Y, Iba T, Tasaka K, Sutou Y, et al. Measurement of endometrial thickness in premenopausal women in office gynecology. *Reproductive Medicine and Biology* 2018:**17**(1):29–35. doi: 10.1002/rmb2.12062.

2. RCOG (Royal College of Obstetricians and Gynaecologists). *Management of endometrial hyperplasia (green-top guideline no. 67).* 2016. Available at: https://www.rcog.org.uk/guidance/browse-all-guidance/green-top-guidelines/management-of-endometrial-hyperplasia-green-top-guideline-no-67.

3. Smith-Bindman R, Weiss E, Feldstein V. How thick is too thick? When endometrial thickness should prompt biopsy in postmenopausal women without vaginal bleeding. *Ultrasound in Obstetrics and Gynaecology* 2004;**24**(5):558–565. doi: 10.1002/uog.1704.

4. RCOG (Royal College of Obstetricians and Gynaecologists). *Ovarian masses in premenopausal women, management of suspected (green-top guideline no. 62),* 2011. Available at: https://www.rcog.org.uk/guidance/browse-all-guidance/green-top-guidelines/ovarian-masses-in-premenopausal-women-management-of-suspected-green-top-guideline-no-62.

5. Brown DL, Dudiak KM, Laing FC. Adnexal masses: US characterization and reporting. *Radiology.* 2010;**254**(2);342–354. doi: 10.1148/radiol.09090552.

5. Huang C, Hong M-K, Ding D-C. A review of ovary torsion. *Tzu Chi Medical Journal* 2017;**29**(3):143–147. doi: 10.4103/tcmj.tcmj_55_17.

6. Van Calster B, Van Hoorde K, Valentin L, Testa AC, Fischerova D, Van Holsbeke C, et al. Evaluating the risk of ovarian cancer before surgery using the ADNEX model to differentiate between benign, borderline, early and advanced stage invasive, and secondary metastatic tumours: Prospective multicentre diagnostic study. *British Medical Journal* 2014:**349**:g5920–g5920. doi: 10.1136/bmj.g5920.

7. Ong CL. The current status of three-dimensional ultrasonography in gynaecology. *Ultrasonography.* 2016;**35**(1):13–24. doi: 10.14366/usg.15043.

8. Siam EM. Pregnancy outcome after hystero-salpingo-contrast-sonography (HyCoSy) versus hysterosalpingography (HSG) using different contrast media. *Middle East Fertility Society Journal* 2011;**16**(4):265–271. doi: 10.1016/j.mefs.2011.05.001.

9. Marci R, Marcucci I, Marcucci AA, Pacini N, Salacone P, Sebastianelli A, et al. Hysterosalpingocontrast sonography (HyCoSy): Evaluation of the pain perception, side effects and complications. *BioMed Central Medical Imaging* 2013;**13**(1)28. doi: 10.1186/1471-2342-13-28.

10. NICE (National Institute for Health and Clinical Excellence). *Fertility problems: Assessment and treatment. Clinical guideline [CG156]*, 2013. Available at: https://www.nice.org.uk/guidance/CG156.

11. Abou-Setta AM, Mansour RT, Al-Inany HG, Aboulghar MM, Aboulghar MA, Serour GI. Among women undergoing embryo transfer, is the probability of pregnancy and live birth improved with ultrasound guidance over clinical touch alone? A systemic review and meta-analysis of prospective randomized trials. *Fertility and Sterility* 2007;**88**(2);333–341. doi: 10.1016/j.fertnstert.2006.11.161.

12. Dickey RP. Doppler ultrasound investigation of uterine and ovarian blood flow in infertility and early pregnancy. *Human Reproduction Update* 1997;**3**(5):467–503. doi: 10.1093/humupd/3.5.467.

13. Strowitzki T, Germeyer A, Popovici R, von Wolff M. The human endometrium as a fertility-determining factor. *Human Reproduction Update* 2006;**12**(5):617–630. doi: 10.1093/humupd/dml033.

14. Chandler TM, Machan LS, Cooperberg PL, Harris AC, Chang SD. Müllerian duct anomalies: From diagnosis to intervention. *British Journal of Radiology* 2009;**82**(984):1034–1042. doi: 10.1259/bjr/99354802.

15. Rock JA. Surgery for anomalies of the Mullerian ducts. In: JD Tompson, JA Rock (eds), *TeLind's operative gynecology*, 9th edn. Philadelphia, PA: JB Lippincott Williams & Wilkins, 2003.

16. Deutch TD, Abuhamad AZ. The role of 3-dimensional ultrasonography and magnetic resonance imaging in the diagnosis of Müllerian duct anomalies: A review of the literature. *Journal of Ultrasound in Medicine*. 2008;**27**(3):413–423. doi: 10.7863/jum.2008.27.3.413.

17. Akhtar MA, Saravelos SH, Li TC, Jayaprakasan K. Reproductive implications and management of congenital uterine anomalies. *British Journal of Obstetrics and Gynaecology*. 2020;**127**(5):e1–e13. doi: 10.1111/1471-0528.15968.

18. Sylvestre C, Child TJ, Tulandi T, Tan SL. A prospective study to evaluate the efficacy of two- and three-dimensional sonohysterography in women with intrauterine lesions. *Fertility and Sterility* 2003;**79**(5):1222–1225. doi: 10.1016/s0015-0282(03)00154-7.

Further reading

D'Angelo A, Amso N (eds). *Ultrasound in assisted reproduction and early pregnancy*. London: CRC Press, 2021.

Rizk BRMB (ed.). *Ultrasonography in reproductive medicine and infertility*. New York: Cambridge University Press, 2003.

Further reading

CHAPTER 8
OBSTETRIC ULTRASOUND

Overview	166
Early pregnancy assessment	169
First trimester	175
Second trimester	179
Third trimester	188
References	194

OVERVIEW

The development of diagnostic ultrasound in the latter half of the twentieth century opened a window on an unseen world and has completely revolutionised the care of the pregnant woman and the fetus. It is the imaging method of choice for screening, diagnosis, intervention and monitoring of pregnancy, and both transabdominal and transvaginal techniques can be used in all three trimesters.

Routine screening scans

There are two routine scans offered in the UK, which are discussed in this chapter:

- The 10 to 14 week scan for dating and assessment.
- The 18 to 21 week scan to check for fetal anomalies and placental site.

Scans for complications

- Known gynaecological conditions.
- Fetal anomalies and non-standard growth patterns requiring monitoring.
- Interventions – chorionic villus sampling (CVS), amniocentesis, cordocentesis, fetal transfusion, shunt placement, membrane lasering or amniotic fluid drainage.
- Situations such as a low-lying placenta or vasa praevia.
- High-risk pregnancies due to either fetal or maternal conditions, including multiple pregnancy, previous preterm delivery, maternal diabetes, hypertension or autoimmune conditions.

Emergency scans

- Hyperemesis in early pregnancy.
- Unexplained pain and/or per vagina bleeding.
- Reduced fetal movements in later pregnancy.
- Suspicion of fetal growth restriction (FGR).
- Absence of detectable fetal heartbeat in the hospital setting.

- Fetal presentation in late pregnancy.
- Spontaneous rupture of membranes.

An early dating scan (**Figure 8.1**) may be performed in particular circumstances, for instance when there have been previous early pregnancy complications, if a termination is requested or there are conditions needing urgent treatment. However, the routine system in the UK is to offer two routine scans, in line with the NHS Fetal Anomaly Screening Programme (NHS FASP).[1] The first of these should be between 11 weeks and 2 days and 14 weeks and 1 day (11^{+2} to 14^{+1} weeks), and the second between 18 weeks and 20 weeks and 6 days (18^{+0} to 20^{+6} weeks) gestation, as calculated by the first scan (**Figures 8.2** and **8.3**). These examinations are described in detail later in this chapter.

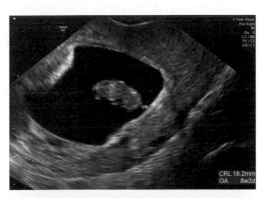

Figure 8.1 A fetus scanned at 8 weeks' gestation, referred via the early pregnancy assessment unit; all was well in this instance.

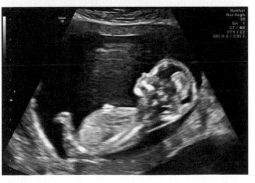

Figure 8.2 A fetus of around 13 weeks' gestation. Although recognisably human at this stage, there is much still to develop internally.

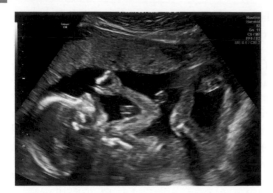

Figure 8.3 At about 19 weeks; the placenta can be seen as the homogeneous grey area in the upper left part of the image.

Fetal measurements are initially undertaken to date the pregnancy; it has been suggested this is best by crown–rump length (CRL) up to 84 mm and then by head circumference (HC) when the CRL is greater than 84 mm.[1,2] Subsequent fetal biometry can then be used to monitor growth and development by comparison with charts of the expected range of measurements. The biometry measurements are inserted into the examination report, allowing visual representations of fetal growth in graphic form. This enables comparison of trends in fetal growth using either population growth charts or customised growth charts for the individual pregnancy, which take into account maternal factors such as height, weight, ethnicity and parity.

Maternity ultrasound services vary greatly between different countries and between different service providers within countries. The UK perspective is provided to highlight what can be achieved within a fully resourced screening and diagnostic service. Although there may be other models available, this is recommended practice where staffing, expertise, equipment, funding and quality assurance programmes allow.

Non-routine obstetric scans, whether for complications or in an emergency situation, should be in accordance with need and adherent to a local protocol. Many women are referred for scans in the third trimester to assess fetal development (**Figure 8.4**). These may include the use of Doppler ultrasound to monitor the blood flow in the uterine, umbilical and fetal middle cerebral and other arteries and in the ductus venosus. Three-dimensional (3D) scanning can be useful when diagnosing complex anomalies and to visualise facial clefts, heart defects and spinal lesions. This aids treatment planning and has vastly improved the prognosis for babies so affected. Three-dimensional and real-time 3D (four-dimensional [4D]) scanning can assist counselling parents when something unexpected has been detected, enabling shared decision-making.

Attention should be given to the woman's privacy and dignity at all times, and the emotional dimension of pregnancy acknowledged.

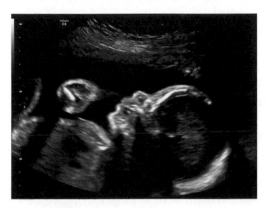

Figure 8.4 A sagittal section of the fetus, showing the face in profile in the third trimester.

EARLY PREGNANCY ASSESSMENT

The suitability of ultrasound as an imaging tool is no better demonstrated than in its use in assessment of pregnancy in the first trimester. The use of two-dimensional (2D) real-time transabdominal transducers (3.5–5 MHz) and the introduction of high-resolution transvaginal transducers (typically at least 7.5 MHz) have allowed visualisation of the developing embryo as early as 5–6 weeks following menstruation. Transvaginal scanning allows much earlier recognition of a normally developing pregnancy, pregnancy failure and ectopic pregnancy, and this is the recommended technique in all cases.[3,4]

Ultrasonic assessment of early pregnancy should be performed in conjunction with blood tests to check the levels of human chorionic gonadotrophin (hCG) – a hormone produced by placental tissue. This is best managed within a dedicated early pregnancy assessment unit (EPAU).

Indications

Ultrasound and in particular transvaginal ultrasound can be used in the first trimester to:

- identify the location of the pregnancy and number of gestation sacs and embryos;
- date the pregnancy;
- assess whether an early pregnancy has a normal appearance or whether the pregnancy has failed;
- assess the pelvis to determine the cause of pain and/or vaginal bleeding.

Patient preparation

When scanning the uterus and ovaries transabdominally, the use of a full bladder is necessary as this allows visualisation of the structures posterior to it. A preliminary survey scan of the pelvis can then be performed. However, in many situations a transvaginal scan will be necessary, and this is carried out with an empty bladder.

A full explanation of the techniques involved must be given to ensure valid, informed consent, either verbally or in writing. During a transabdominal scan the lower abdomen needs to be exposed to the symphysis pubis; however, for a transvaginal scan, removal of all garments below the waist is required. Use of a chaperone is advised.

A suitable single-use cover must be used over the probe and gloves worn by the operator. If the probe cover and gloves contain latex, the woman should be checked for latex allergy and vinyl alternatives used if necessary. Gel is applied to the probe before covering to exclude air between the surface of the probe and the cover that might inhibit transmission of the ultrasound. Sterile lubricant is applied to the outer surface of the cover. Before and after use, the probe must be disinfected according to the manufacturer's guidelines, and this process documented to provide a clear audit trail.

Imaging procedure

The examination is carried out with the woman in a supine position for both a transabdominal and a transvaginal scan. For transabdominal ultrasound, gel is applied to the pelvic area and the long axis of the transducer is placed in the midline above the symphysis pubis. A systematic scan of the uterus and adnexae is carried out in both longitudinal and transverse planes as an initial assessment of the entire pelvic area. Subsequent targeted views using a zoom facility or a selected high-resolution portion of the image allow a thorough examination of any specific areas of interest, such as an early gestation sac, a developing embryo or a definite or suspected ectopic pregnancy.

Due to the small size of the structures to be visualised, a transvaginal scan is recommended. As the transducer is in closer proximity to the structures being examined, a higher frequency can be used and this gives better resolution. If a transvaginal scan is required, the use of a cushion to lift the pelvis off the couch is advantageous, or a couch with a removable lower section may also be used to improve access and reduce the risk of work-related musculoskeletal injury to the operator. The probe, once in position, can be angled and rotated in order to visualise the uterus, ovaries and surrounding area. Good, clear communication is required to ensure that the woman understands what will happen during the scan and knows that she can ask for the examination to stop at any point.

The use of any sort of Doppler ultrasound should be avoided in the first trimester, especially when using transvaginal scanning because there is a potential for heating, which could affect the vulnerable process of organogenesis.[5] M mode is a lower energy alternative that is useful for confirmation of the fetal heartbeat.[6]

Image analysis

The transabdominal scan in **Figure 8.5** shows the maternal bladder lying anterior to an anteverted uterus. Within the thickened endometrium at the fundus of the uterus is a small, well-defined, fluid-filled area, which is an early gestation sac. Structures within the gestation sac may be visible only if a transvaginal scan is performed.[7] The transvaginal scan in **Figure 8.6** also shows an anteverted uterus with a pregnancy at around the same stage. The gestation sac is well defined, with a bright border; this is a decidual reaction and is typical of an early pregnancy.

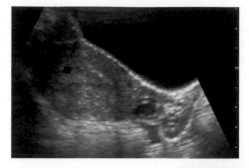

Figure 8.5 (left) Trans-abdominal scan, showing an early gestation sac at the fundus of the uterus.

Figure 8.6 (right) Transvaginal scan in a different patient, showing an early gestation sac at the fundus of the uterus.

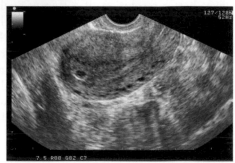

The transvaginal scan in **Figure 8.7** demonstrates a pregnancy of around 5–6 weeks. The yolk sac is visible as a ring-like structure within the gestation sac and is the primary maternal–fetal transport system before the establishment of placental circulation, so these appearances are strongly suggestive of a developing pregnancy.[7,8]

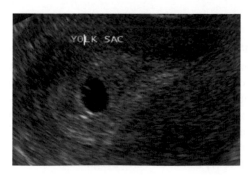

Figure 8.7 Gestation sac of 5–6 weeks containing a yolk sac.

A pregnancy of approximately 6–7 weeks gestation, scanned trans-vaginally is shown in **Figure 8.8**. Within the gestation sac can be seen both the developing embryo to the left and the yolk sac to the right, connected by the vitelline duct (yolk stalk). Cardiac pulsations will be readily seen at this stage on real-time ultrasound.[9] The embryo measures around 6–7 mm at this stage. A thick trophoblastic rim is seen surrounding the sac, the beginning of placental development.

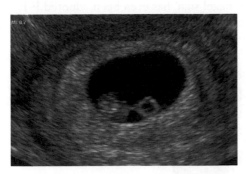

Figure 8.8 Gestation sac containing an embryo and yolk sac.

A transvaginal image of a monochorionic twin pregnancy is seen in **Figure 8.9**, where both embryos are within one gestation sac. A dichorionic twin pregnancy would be seen as two separate gestation sacs, each containing an embryo and yolk sac. It is important to determine the chorionicity in the first trimester, as monochorionic twins have a greater risk of complications throughout the pregnancy.[10,11]

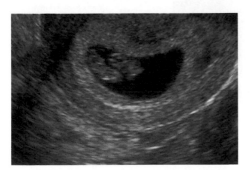

Figure 8.9 A twin pregnancy.

The transabdominal scan with a maternal full bladder in **Figure 8.10** shows an ectopic pregnancy. Above the highest point of the uterus, a ring-like structure is clearly visible; this is the ectopic pregnancy. **Figure 8.11** is a transvaginal scan of an ectopic pregnancy. The right ovary can be seen in the centre of the image, and adjacent to this the ectopic pregnancy can be seen laterally as a ring-like structure towards the left-hand side of the image. Ectopic pregnancies are sometimes described as doughnut like, and the term 'bagel sign' has even been adopted.[12] It is important to look for the presence of fluid in the pelvis as this can be a sign of bleeding, indicating rupture of the fallopian tube.[4]

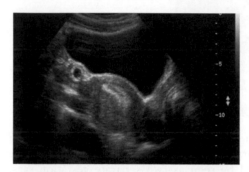

Figure 8.10 An ectopic pregnancy.

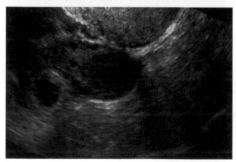

Figure 8.11 Right adnexal ectopic pregnancy.

FIRST TRIMESTER

In England, the NHS FASP has made good progress in standardising ultrasonic imaging in the first and second trimesters of pregnancy. Similar programmes are in place in Scotland and Wales.

Indications

Ultrasound is offered routinely in the first trimester for:
- examination of pelvic adnexa for any related gynaecological problems;
- checking that the fetal heart pulsations are present;
- confirming the site of pregnancy – intrauterine or extrauterine;
- dating of pregnancy (estimation of gestational age); this is crucial for the timing of particular antenatal tests and for optimising delivery time;
- screening tests, particularly the measurement of the nuchal translucency as part of the combined screening test; this test gives a result suggesting the chance of the baby having Down's syndrome, Edwards' syndrome and Patau's syndrome;[1]
- diagnosis or exclusion of a number of major structural abnormalities;
- guidance for invasive procedures such as CVS;
- establishing a baseline for subsequent monitoring of fetal growth;
- detection and assessment of multiple pregnancy.

Patient preparation

The preparation for transabdominal ultrasound is generally to drink 900 ml (a pint and a half) of clear fluid an hour before the examination in order to fill the maternal urinary bladder. This provides an acoustic window to allow visualisation of pelvic structures and displace bowel gas.

A full explanation of the procedure and the reasons for the examination must be given to the patient, and the date of the last normal menstrual period and any relevant medical and obstetric history should be noted.

After the procedure, the gel should be wiped from the abdomen and probe. The probe should be cleaned according to the manufacturer's instructions. An explanation of the findings on completion of the examination is usual.

Imaging procedure

Transabdominal ultrasound is the main method of assessing the fetus for first trimester screening. Transvaginal ultrasound may also be used, as described in this chapter in the section on 'Early pregnancy assessment'.

Longitudinal images are obtained by holding the probe vertically in the midline sagittal plane, initially superior to the symphysis pubis. Parasagittal sections are then obtained by sliding the probe in a continuous scanning action to each side of the lower abdomen and pelvis. The probe is then rotated through 90° and transverse images of the lower abdomen are achieved, starting superior to the symphysis pubis and sliding the probe cranially with a continuous scanning action.

Additional oblique scan sections are required to complete the examination along with rocking and angling movements of the probe as appropriate to obtain the required sections to demonstrate the maternal pelvic organs and assess for any incidental gynaecological pathology. The sonographer must also evaluate the siting of the pregnancy, fetal position, cardiac pulsations, biometry, appearances of fetal structure in relation to the gestational age, the number of fetuses present and the liquor volume.

Accurate fetal biometry in the first trimester is essential to set the parameters for any subsequent investigations and interventions, including optimising the timing of delivery. The fetal CRL is measured to establish gestational age, although by the end of the first trimester the HC may be used.[13]

The fetal nuchal translucency (NT) is also measured at the time of the first trimester scan if the combined screening test for Down's, Edwards' and Patau's syndromes is required.[1] For the purposes of combined screening, the CRL and NT must be measured within the specific time frame of 11[+2] to 14[+1] weeks, defined as when the CRL is between 45 mm and 84 mm.[1] It is crucial for the CRL to be measured accurately to ensure optimal test performance for women choosing to be screened for the three syndromes. The NT measurement is used by the laboratory in conjunction with maternal blood serum biochemical markers and other data to calculate the chance of the fetus having Down's, Edwards' or Patau's syndrome. Women who have a combined screening test result suggesting a higher chance of their baby having one of the three syndromes are offered invasive diagnostic testing. This may be by amniocentesis, when some of the amniotic fluid containing fetal cells is extracted under ultrasound control and sent for analysis, or by CVS, when a sample of cells is taken from placental tissue. Cell-free non-invasive prenatal testing (cfNIPT), in which tiny amounts of fetal DNA that have crossed the placental barrier can be examined in a maternal blood sample,[13] is another means of cytogenetic testing being offered when the chance of Down's, Edwards' or Patau's syndrome is between 1:2 and 1:150.[14]

Under optimum conditions, it may be possible to assess the first trimester fetus for structural anomalies and the NHS FASP is exploring practice in this direction to enable earlier intervention if required. For instance, visualisation of the normal fetal stomach excludes upper gut atresia and fluid in the fetal bladder can be taken as confirmation of renal function. Current and future developments in both imaging technology and protocols are expected to shift elements of the second trimester screening for structural anomalies into the first trimester.

Image analysis

The CRL is the length of the fetus from the crown (top of the head) to the rump (base of the bottom). There is a high degree of correlation between fetal length and gestational age because it is a linear measurement and in the earlier stages of pregnancy is less likely to be influenced by individual characteristics. If performed correctly it is the most accurate parameter for assessment of gestational age.

An ideal section to measure the CRL is a midline sagittal section with the fetus horizontal on the screen, so that the line between the crown and the rump is at 90° to the ultrasound beam (**Figure 8.12**). The image should be magnified to clearly demonstrate the whole length from the crown to the rump. Electronic callipers are used to measure the un-flexed length in which the end points of the crown and the rump are clearly defined.

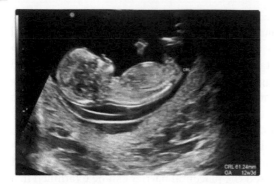

Figure 8.12 Crown–rump length measurement (61.2 mm) towards the end of the first trimester, giving a gestational age of 12 weeks and 3 days.

The NT can be defined as the subcutaneous collection of fluid under the skin of the fetal neck. The NT measurement is obtained from a midline sagittal section with the fetus horizontal on the screen (**Figures 8.13** and **8.14**).

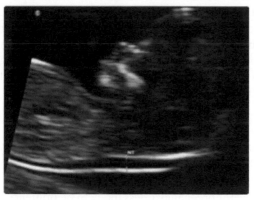

Figure 8.13 Nuchal translucency (NT) measurement.

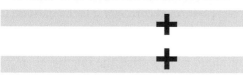

Figure 8.14 Fetal Anomaly Screening Programme diagram of calliper placement for nuchal translucency measurement.

An NT measurement is demonstrated in **Figure 8.13**. The widest part of the NT, the fluid area (which appears black), is measured. Careful placement of the callipers is essential, to ensure accurate calculation of the chance of the three syndromes is made. Measurements should be taken with the inner border of the horizontal line of the callipers placed ON the line that defines the NT thickness. The crossbar of the calliper should be such that it is hardly visible as it merges with the white line of the border, not in the nuchal fluid. **Figure 8.14** illustrates the correct calliper placement for NT measurement, where the two blue lines represent the fetal tissue borders, which show as white lines in the sonogram of **Figure 8.13**.

SECOND TRIMESTER

Transabdominal real time 2D ultrasound is the imaging method of choice for the second trimester of pregnancy and has completely revolutionised antenatal care.

In the second trimester of pregnancy, it is possible to undertake an extensive survey for fetal anomalies, which may be abnormalities in themselves or suggestive of underlying conditions. In England, this is based on standards and guidelines from the NHS FASP, in accordance with the National Screening Committee's criteria for an effective screening programme,[1] with similar programmes in Scotland and Wales.

Indications

The main indication for an ultrasound scan in the second trimester is the 20-week screening scan, which is offered to all pregnant women and usually undertaken between 18^{+0} and 20^{+6} weeks' gestation, ideally as calculated by the first trimester dating scan.[1,15] In the absence of a prior dating scan, the HC can be used to establish gestational age.

Scans may also be performed in the second trimester to localise the fetus, placenta and cord for amniocentesis, and to perform cordocentesis for diagnostic or therapeutic percutaneous umbilical blood sampling (PUBS).

Patient preparation

For transabdominal ultrasound, a full bladder is preferred in order to displace bowel gas and provide an acoustic window, allowing better visualisation of pelvic structures. The woman lies supine on the examination couch and coupling gel is applied to the bare lower abdomen.

Written and verbal information should be offered, with time for questions and maternal consent obtained before the scan is undertaken. Information must include a full explanation of the procedure and its benefits and limitations, along with the implications of possible unexpected findings.

Imaging procedure

Using a curvilinear probe with a transducer frequency range of 3.5–5 MHz for maximum detail, an initial survey scan will examine the uterus and adnexae for any obvious gynaecological pathology, establish the number of fetuses present and check for heartbeat and movements.

The procedure is to obtain longitudinal images by holding the probe in the midline sagittal plane initially superior to the symphysis pubis. Parasagittal sections are then obtained by sliding the probe in a continuous scanning action to each side of the lower abdomen and pelvis. The probe is then rotated through 90° and transverse axial images are achieved to cover the lower abdomen from the symphysis pubis to the fundus of the uterus. This will reveal the fetal position and enable the sonographer to work out the fetal lie, including the presenting part, which way the fetus is facing, and crucially its laterality (which are its left and right sides). This is important in checking situs, in other words that the heart and intra-abdominal organs are correctly sited, as well as ensuring that the limbs of both sides are examined. The placental site and liquor volume are also subjectively assessed. If the placenta is close to or abutting the internal os (the opening to the cervix), a measurement can be taken from the leading edge of the placenta to the internal os. The cervical canal and the internal os can also be checked to ensure that there is no cervical shortening or opening of the internal os, which might suggest an increased chance of preterm delivery.

From this point onwards, the probe is aligned with longitudinal and transverse sections of the fetus rather than the mother, to enable detailed examination of key fetal anatomy in two planes. Although the fetus at this stage of development is highly mobile, the sonographer will be able to track the movement and maintain awareness of position and situs. The 20-week scan is one of the most intricate and crucial examinations that can be performed, and the number of checks to be made in such a small area of high mobility demands a systematic examination and the utmost concentration. If the pregnancy is a twin or higher multiple pregnancy, each fetus must be identified and examined separately to ensure that no part is missed.

Measurements taken and recorded are the fetal HC, abdominal circumference (AC) and femur length (FL). These are compared with the normal range of values at the calculated gestational age to determine the fetal growth rate, as aberrations in growth may be indicative of further conditions.

Once the various regions of interest have been identified, examined and measured where appropriate, it is usual to demonstrate the key points to the mother and support person, if present, and often produce images of the more recognisable sections as 'keepsakes'.

Image analysis

An ultrasound 'base menu' has been devised in accordance with the NHS FASP guidelines, and there are specific anatomical sections to be recorded (**Figures 8.15–8.28**, reproduced by kind permission of the NHS FASP). These include the recommended measurements for assessment of fetal growth and development (**Figures 8.15–8.18** and **8.21–8.24**).

Figures 8.15 and **8.16** show an axial section of the fetal head, demonstrating the midline echo, cavum septum pellucidum, choroid plexus and posterior horn of the lateral ventricular atrium (VA). These landmarks within the fetal brain verify that this is the correct section for biometry, and electronic callipers can be seen measuring the fetal HC and VA. The former is used as a measure of fetal growth and development or for dating if there is no prior dating scan, and the latter is used to assess ventricular size. A normal VA measurement should be less than 10 mm.[1]

Moving slightly lower in the posterior region of the fetal head, by tilting the probe from the axial measurement section, enables

Figure 8.15
Second trimester
head circumference
and ventricular atrium
measurements.

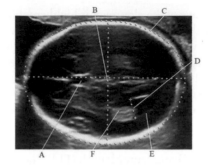

Figure 8.16
Diagram to illustrate
anatomy and calliper
placement. HC, head
circumference; VA,
ventricular atrium.

B Mid-line echo

C HC measurement

D Measurement of
the VA, inner edge
to inner edge of
the ventricular
walls at its widest
part, and aligned
perpendicular to
the long axis of
the atrium

A Cavum septum
pellucidum

F Choroid plexus

E Posterior horn
of ventricle

demonstration of the posterior fossa (**Figures 8.17** and **8.18**). Electronic callipers can be seen measuring the transcerebellar diameter (TCD) and nuchal fold (NF). A normally configured posterior fossa at this stage suggests normal brain and spinal cord development thus far.[16]

The fetal lips and nasal tip in an oblique coronal section are demonstrated in **Figures 8.19** and **8.20**, enabling continuity of the soft-tissue lines to be checked. Discontinuities may be indicative of a cleft lip or palate, which responds very well to early corrective surgery. Failure to diagnose or to treat this at an early stage may lead to serious feeding difficulties as well as future disfigurement,[17] although an isolated cleft palate can be difficult to diagnose.

Figure 8.17 The trans-cerebellar diameter and nuchal fold.

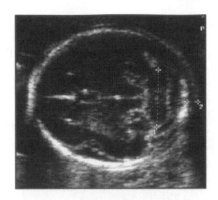

Figure 8.18 Corresponding diagram to show calliper placement. NF, nuchal fold; TCD, transcerebellar diameter.

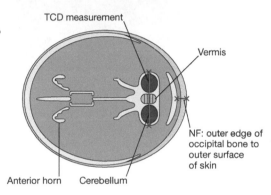

TCD measurement

Vermis

NF: outer edge of occipital bone to outer surface of skin

Anterior horn   Cerebellum

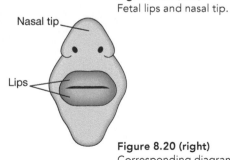

Figure 8.19 (left) Fetal lips and nasal tip.

Nasal tip

Lips

Figure 8.20 (right) Corresponding diagram to identify the features.

183

An axial section of the fetal abdomen, including the stomach and liver, is shown in **Figures 8.21** and **8.22**. Electronic callipers can be seen measuring the fetal AC. Visualisation of fluid in the fetal stomach suggests that swallowing is taking place.

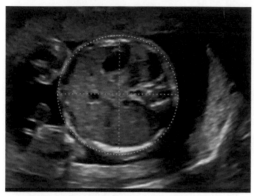

Figure 8.21 Second trimester abdominal circumference measurement.

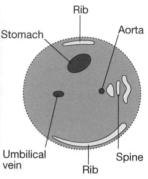

Figure 8.22 Diagram to show landmarks and calliper placement.

The FL with measurement callipers is demonstrated in **Figures 8.23** and **8.24**. Any discrepancy at this stage may suggest complications with growth or a type of skeletal dysplasia and can be investigated or monitored. NHS FASP[1] recommend reporting any FL measurement measuring 'significantly' less than the 5th centile for gestational age.

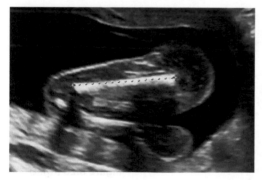

Figure 8.23 Second trimester femur length measurement.

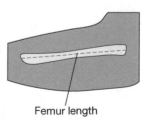

Figure 8.24 Diagram of calliper placement for femur length measurement.

A sagittal section of the fetal spine, showing complete skin covering in the midline, is shown in **Figures 8.25** and **8.26**. This can exclude an open neural tube defect such as spina bifida. The most common location for spina bifida is in the lumbosacral region. If the fetus is in the supine position, it is often beneficial to wait for it to turn to see the spine clearly. The fetal bladder and aorta can also be seen in **Figure 8.25**. The fetal bladder can only be filled by anterograde flow, so its visualisation confirms renal function.

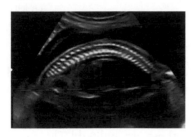

Figure 8.25 Fetal sagittal section showing the spine longitudinally.

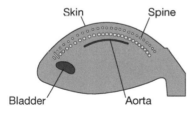

Figure 8.26 Illustration of the skin covering the spine in the midline.

Checking the heart, outflow tracts and connections is a complicated process, during which the sonographer must use considerable deftness to acquire several precise sections. One of these is illustrated in **Figure 8.27**, the four-chamber view, with the anatomy detailed in the accompanying diagram of **Figure 8.28**. The heart itself is only thumbnail sized at this stage and, because many defects are relatively small, and the circulation changes with the first breaths of life, not all defects may be apparent; some remain diagnosable only postnatally. Further images can be seen in the NHS FASP handbook.[1]

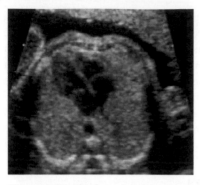

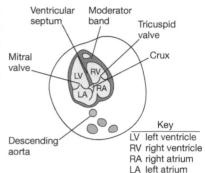

Figure 8.27 The four-chamber view of the fetal heart.

Figure 8.28 Anatomical features within the four-chamber view.

Other fetal anatomy checked during the assessment includes the limbs, abdominal organs and chest, including the situs and laterality.

Eleven specific conditions have been agreed as detectable by the NHS FASP, and the detection rates of these are audited.[1] These conditions are:
- anencephaly;
- spina bifida;
- cleft lip;
- congenital diaphragmatic hernia;
- gastroschisis;
- exomphalos;
- congenital heart disease;
- bilateral renal agenesis;
- lethal skeletal dysplasia;
- Edwards' syndrome (trisomy 18);
- Patau's syndrome (trisomy 13).

In the event of untoward findings, further images would be recorded as appropriate and Doppler may be used. The findings would then be discussed with the mother and her support person, if present. Follow-up scans are often required, and sometimes magnetic resonance imaging (MRI) is offered or invasive procedures to obtain fetal cells for a definitive diagnosis. After this there are differing courses of action, depending on the choice of the mother, varying from no intervention to termination for the severest abnormalities that may be incompatible with life. In general, the NHS FASP has resulted in the finding of many anomalies, enabling treatment at an early stage and sometimes even in utero surgery. The pregnant woman may continue to be cared for locally or may be referred to a regional fetal medicine unit if further investigation, diagnosis, monitoring or intervention is called for.

Once the assessment of the fetus is complete, it is common to show the parents a profile and provide a 'keepsake' image if possible. **Figure 8.29** is a longitudinal midline section of the fetus, showing the body and face in profile, with one of the lower limbs visible at the extreme left of the image. Anterior to the fetal face, a few sections of the umbilical cord are visible. This section is also useful to assess the normality of the fetal profile, assessing the alignment of the forehead, nose and chin, along with the integrity of the anterior chest and abdominal wall.

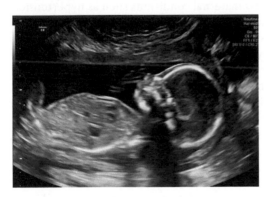

Figure 8.29 A 'keepsake' image at around 20 weeks.

THIRD TRIMESTER

Ultrasound is not used routinely in the third trimester in low-risk pregnancies; however, it is used in assessing high-risk pregnancies such as multiple pregnancy and pregnancies with complications. Standard fetal biometry measurements are taken of the fetus in addition to assessing the amniotic fluid levels, placental position and blood flow to and from the fetus using Doppler.

Indications

Scans are often performed in the third trimester to assess fetal growth and liquor, particularly if the uterine fundus measures 'small for dates' on palpation, if there is a history of pregnancy problems or if the pregnancy is complicated by maternal conditions such as hypertension, diabetes, sickle cell disease or maternal obesity. All multiple pregnancies have regular third trimester growth scans. Continuing pregnancies in which a fetal abnormality has been detected are often assessed in the third trimester. Assessment of the pregnancy may also be carried out if the placenta is covering the internal os at the second trimester anomaly scan; if there is uncertainty about the fetal lie near to term, or for reassurance following injury or bleeding.

In some pregnancies, a single third trimester scan may be performed, whereas in others, serial growth scans are carried out every 3–4 weeks. If the pregnancy is showing signs of further complications such as FGR, then scans for amniotic fluid volume and assessment of blood flow using Doppler ultrasound may be performed. Growth scans to assess changes in fetal growth profile or estimated fetal weight should normally be carried out at least 3 weeks apart.[18]

Patient preparation

Most third trimester scans are carried out transabdominally. As the fetus is surrounded with amniotic fluid, which acts as an acoustic window, no preparation is required. Occasionally a transvaginal scan (TVS) is needed, particularly for placental localisation or for measurement of cervical length. An empty bladder is required for the TVS, and consent, infection control and attention to privacy and dignity are observed as described elsewhere. An awareness of the emotional impact of the examination is essential, as most third trimester scans are carried out on high-risk pregnancies. Following the scan the gel is removed and the results of the examination explained to the parents. Demonstrating the growth on the graph is helpful for understanding.

Imaging procedure

Usually, the mother lies in the supine position on the couch, although as pregnancy progresses this can lead to supine hypotension. This occurs when the fetus presses on the inferior vena cava causing low blood pressure, which can lead to dizziness and fainting. Turning the mother slightly on to her side, using pillows or cushions for support, alleviates the symptoms.

Initially the internal os is visualised, using a curvilinear array transducer with a frequency of 2.5–5 MHz longitudinally in the midline, just above the symphysis pubis. Next, the fetal lie and location of the placenta are assessed, to determine their relative relationship. Near to term, it is important to determine whether the fetus is cephalic (head down) or breech. Breech (bottom first) deliveries are more complicated and the midwife needs to know which part of the fetus is presenting. Footling breech (feet presenting) increases the risk of cord prolapse, leading to a reduction in the oxygen supply to the fetus. The placental site is also important, as a placenta completely covering the internal os requires a caesarean section to prevent haemorrhage and neonatal death.

The fetus is assessed in detail, again reviewing the anatomy. Measurements for growth are taken, including the HC, AC and FL (**Figures 8.30** to **8.32**).

Image analysis

An axial section through the fetal head in **Figure 8.30** demonstrates the oval shape, intact skull, symmetrical hemispheres of the brain, the cavum septum pellucidum (hypoechoic 'box' in the midline near the front of the head) and the lateral ventricles. The dotted line shows the circumference (HC) measurement.

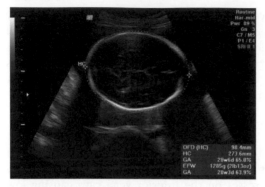

Figure 8.30 Third trimester HC measurement. EFW, estimate fetal weight; GA, gestational age; HC, head circumference; OFD, occipitofrontal diameter.

An axial section through the fetal abdomen, demonstrating the rounded shape, a portion of the fluid-filled stomach and the central section of the umbilical vein is shown in **Figure 8.31**, approximately one-third of the way in from the anterior abdominal wall. The dotted line shows the circumference (AC).

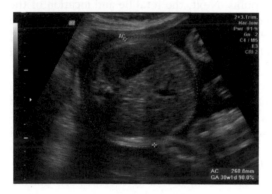

Figure 8.31 Third trimester abdominal circumference (AC) measurement.

The probe should be angled to demonstrate the full length of the femoral shaft horizontally. Calliper placement on each end for measurement is demonstrated in **Figure 8.32**.

The fetal measurements are plotted on to graphs to demonstrate the growth profile of the individual fetus compared with pre-plotted lines based on statistics for the population group, usually nationally determined,[13] as in **Figure 8.33**. This shows the normal range for measurements. Measurements above the 90th centile are large for the

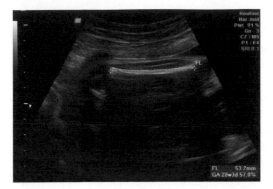

Figure 8.32 Third trimester femur length (FL) measurement.

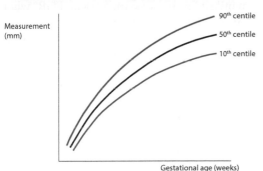

Figure 8.33 Growth graph demonstrating the 90th, 50th and 10th centiles.

gestational age and measurements below the 10th centile suggest that the fetus is small for gestational age. Each fetus has an expected growth potential, dependent on the baseline growth measurements taken earlier in pregnancy and other factors such as maternal height, weight, ethnicity and birth weight of previous pregnancies. Individualised growth charts are more commonly used now to account for these factors, although consensus has not been reached on which is optimal.

If growth is less than expected, for example below the 10th centile for the gestational age, this is known as FGR.[18] In some cases, the measurement may be within the normal centile range, but a much lower centile than previous scans, for instance growth at the 80th centile reducing to growth along the 30th centile.[19] By comparing the growth for both the HC and the AC, FGR may be classified as symmetrical or asymmetrical.

If the HC and AC are both less than expected, this is said to be symmetrical FGR, which is linked to many factors including chromosomal abnormalities, maternal malnutrition, smoking and drug taking.

If the AC growth profile is less than anticipated, but the HC is normal, this is said to be asymmetrical FGR. This is often caused by placental insufficiency, and the fetus tries to compensate for this by increasing blood supply to the fetal brain, myocardium and adrenal glands, at the expense of other organs. This leads to the 'brain-sparing' effect, causing the HC:AC growth discrepancy.

However, the early stages of symmetrical FGR may appear to be asymmetrical as physiological compensation occurs, and prolonged asymmetrical FGR may manifest as more symmetrical FGR when these mechanisms fail, so this situation is far from clear cut.

In any case of suspected growth restriction, the sonographer should check for any visible coexistent condition. The liquor volume should also be checked, as there can often be associated oligohydramnios (reduced amniotic fluid). The amniotic fluid or liquor volume can be

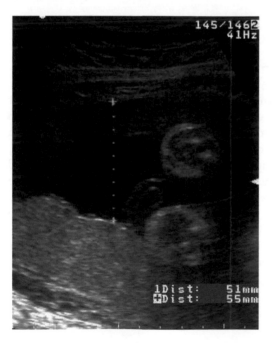

145/1462
41Hz

1Dist: 51mm
⊕Dist: 55mm

Figure 8.34 Measurement of a normal pool of amniotic fluid.

estimated by measurement of the deepest clear pool of amniotic fluid, as seen in **Figure 8.34**. Normal range is 2–8 cm.[19] Less than 2 cm would suggest oligohydramnios, which is common in FGR. The placenta can be seen posteriorly on this image.

Another very useful indicator of fetal health is assessment of the blood flow in the umbilical artery using Doppler ultrasound (**Figure 8.35**). The normal waveform shows pulsatile and unidirectional flow throughout the fetal cardiac cycle, indicative of good fetal cardiac output. If there is compromised cardiac output or increased placental resistance, the end-diastolic flow becomes reduced, absent and ultimately reversed. Point A represents the peak systolic velocity and point B the end-diastolic velocity. Other vessels can be assessed, such as the middle cerebral artery, to determine the severity of FGR and redistribution of blood flow.[19] This information is used to manage the timing of delivery.[18]

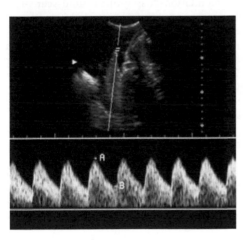

Figure 8.35 Normal spectral Doppler waveform of the umbilical artery.

An estimate of the fetal weight can be calculated using the biparietal diameter, HC, AC and FL measurements, and this may also contribute to the management of delivery. In some cases, growth may be above that expected, or macrosomia, which also needs monitoring, as delivery of a large baby can lead to complications such as shoulder dystocia.

REFERENCES

1. PHE (Public Health England). *Guidance. NHS fetal anomaly screening programme handbook*, 2021. https://www.gov.uk/government/publications/fetal-anomaly-screening-programme-handbook.

2. Chudleigh T, Loughna P, Evans T. A practical solution to combining dating and screening for Down's syndrome. *Ultrasound* 2011;**19**(3):154–157. doi: 10.1258/ult.2011.011028.

3. RCOG (Royal College of Obstetricians and Gynaecologists). *Early pregnancy loss, management (green-top guideline no. 25)*, 2006. Available at: https://www.rcog.org.uk/en/guidelines-research-services/guidelines/gtg25.

4. NICE (National Institute for Health and Care Excellence). *Ectopic pregnancy and miscarriage: diagnosis and initial management. NICE guideline [NG126]*, 2019. Available at: https://www.nice.org.uk/guidance/ng126/chapter/Recommendations#using-ultrasound-scans-for-diagnosis-of-tubal-ectopic-pregnancy.

5. Salvesen K, Lees C, Abramowicz J, Brezinka C, Ter Haar G, Maršál K, et al. Board of International Society of Ultrasound in Obstetrics and Gynecology (ISUOG). ISUOG statement on the safe use of Doppler in the 11 to 13+6-week fetal ultrasound examination. *Ultrasound in Obsetrics and Gynecology* 2011;**37**(6):628. doi: 10.1002/uog.9026.

6. RCOG (Royal College of Obstetricians and Gynaecologists). *Ultrasound from conception to 10^{+0} weeks of gestation (scientific impact paper no. 49)*, 2015. Available at: https://www.rcog.org.uk/guidance/browse-all-guidance/scientific-impact-papers/ultrasound-from-conception-to-10plus0-weeks-of-gestation-scientific-impact-paper-no-49.

7. Rodgers SK, Chang C, DeBardeleben JT, Horrow MM. Normal and abnormal US findings in early first-trimester pregnancy: Review of the Society of Radiologists in Ultrasound 2012 consensus panel recommendations. *Radiographics* 2015;**35**(7):2135–2148. doi: 10.1148/rg.2015150092.

8. Lindsay DJ, Lovett IS, Lyons EA, Levi CS, Zheng XH, Holt SC, et al. Yolk sac diameter and shape at endovaginal US: Predictors of pregnancy outcome in the first trimester. *Radiology* 1992;**183**(1):115–118. doi: 10.1148/radiology.183.1.1549656.

9. Doubilet PM, Benson CB, Bourne T, Blaivas M. Diagnostic criteria for nonviable pregnancy early in the first trimester. *New England Journal of Medicine* 2013;**369**(15):1443–1451. doi: 10.1056/NEJMra1302417.

10. Khalil A, Rodgers M, Baschat A, Bhide A, Gratacos E, Hecher K, et al. ISUOG Practice guidelines: Role of ultrasound in twin pregnancy. *Ultrasound in Obstetrics and Gynecology* 2016;**47**(2):247–263. doi: 10.1002/uog.15821.

11. NICE (National Institute for Health and Care Excellence). *Twin and triplet pregnancy. NICE guideline [NG137]*, 2019. Available at: https://www.nice.org.uk/guidance/ng137/chapter/Recommendations#fetal-complications.

12. Goldstein S, Timor-Tritsch IE. *Ultrasound in gynaecology.* New York: Churchill Livingstone, 1995.

13. Chitty LS. Use of cell-free DNA to screen for Down's syndrome. *New England Journal of Medicine* 2015;**372**(17):1666–1667. doi: 10.1056/NEJMe1502441.

13. Loughna P, Chitty L, Evans T, Chudleigh T. Ultrasound fetal size and dating: Charts recommended for clinical obstetric practice. *Ultrasound* 2009;**17**(3):161–167. doi: 10.1179/174313409X448543.

14. PHE (Public Health England). *Guidance. Screening for Down's syndrome, Edwards' syndrome and Patau's syndrome: NIPT*, 2021. Available at: https://www.gov.uk/government/publications/screening-for-downs-syndrome-edwards-syndrome-and-pataus-syndrome-non-invasive-prenatal-testing-nipt/screening-for-downs-syndrome-edwards-syndrome-and-pataus-syndrome-nipt.

15. NHS Scotland. *National protocols. Programme: Fetal anomaly and Down's syndrome screening.* Edinburgh: NHS Scotland, 2015:1–58. Available at: https://www.pnsd.scot.nhs.uk/wp-content/2015-Fetal-Anomaly-and-Downs-Syndrome-Screening-Protocols-v-1.pdf.

16. Van den Hof MC, Nicolaides KH, Campbell J, Campbell S. Evaluation of the lemon and banana signs in one hundred thirty fetuses with open spina bifida. *American Journal of Obstetrics and Gynecology* 1990;**162**(2): 322–327. doi: 10.1016/0002-9378(90)90378-k.

17. Masarei AG, Sell D, Habel A, Mars M, Sommerlad BC, Wade A. The nature of feeding in infants with unrepaired cleft lip and/or palate compared with healthy noncleft infants. *Cleft Palate-Craniofacial Journal* 2007;**44**(3):321–328. doi: 10.1597/05-185.

18. RCOG (Royal College of Obstetricians and Gynaecologists). *Small-for-gestational-age fetus investigation and management (green-top guideline no. 31)*, 2013. Available at: https://www.rcog.org.uk/guidance/browse-all-guidance/green-top-guidelines/small-for-gestational-age-fetus-investigation-and-management-green-top-guideline-no-31.

19. BMUS 3rd trimester special interest group. Professional guidance for fetal growth scans performed after 23 weeks of gestation. 2022. https://www.bmus.org/policies-statements-guidelines/professional-guidance/guidance-pages/professional-guidance-for-fetal-growth-scans-performed-after-23-weeks-of-gestation.

CHAPTER 9

BREAST ULTRASOUND

Greyscale, Doppler and contrast-enhanced ultrasound (CEUS)   198
Elastography   204
Volume scanning   206
References   209

GREYSCALE, DOPPLER AND CONTRAST-ENHANCED ULTRASOUND (CEUS)

Breast ultrasound imaging is performed with high-frequency transducers to produce dynamic examinations of all types of breast tissues. It is used as the preferred imaging modality in younger women (<40 years old) in the triple assessment of breast symptoms alongside clinical palpation and pathological assessment.[1,2] In the older woman, it is used as an adjuvant to other imaging modalities, especially mammography. Ultrasound can assess the size, shape, outline and echotexture of lesions.

Colourflow or power Doppler and CEUS can be used to assess the vascularity both within masses and in the surrounding tissue. Increased blood flow within a mass may represent neovascularisation. This feature is one that is associated with most actively growing malignant breast cancers and can help in the differential diagnosis of malignancy, although rapidly growing benign masses can also exhibit increased vascularity.[3]

The dynamic nature of breast ultrasound enables accurate real-time tissue sampling of such suspicious masses for pathological assessment.

Indications

The clinical findings of a new palpable lump may raise the suspicion of breast cancer. Mammograms, though very sensitive for demonstrating lesions, lack the specificity of breast ultrasound. The younger breast is generally very dense and may require higher doses of ionising radiation (X-rays) to penetrate the dense background to produce an adequate, diagnostic mammogram. Symptomatic breast lumps can therefore be examined by ultrasound without the use of ionising radiation in the younger woman.

The National Health Service Breast Screening Programme (NHSBSP) suggests that ultrasound should not be used to screen the asymptomatic breast, as it lacks the sensitivity of mammography.[4,5] However, for women recalled following a mammographic anomaly, ultrasound is a component of the triple assessment procedure.[1]

Patient preparation

No physical patient preparation is required for breast ultrasound. The probe and other equipment are cleaned between patients using manufacturer-approved processes, and appropriate hand hygiene is observed as per local protocol.

After an explanation of the procedure, verbal consent should be obtained before beginning the scan. Dignity for the patient can be maintained by minimal exposure of the breast, with disposable coverings on the contralateral breast. Only essential people should be present; this may include a chaperone.

If there is a chance of an invasive procedure, such as a biopsy or fine-needle aspiration (FNA) being performed during the examination, sterile gel should be used for the whole examination, to reduce the risk of infection.[6]

Post-examination, the patient should be made aware of the local arrangements for obtaining the results of the examination. In some cases, patients are seen in one-stop clinics, where they receive the results of the ultrasound scan and any other investigations, such as mammogram and FNA, at the same time. This enables early discussion of the findings and potential management options with a clinician.

Imaging procedure

A pillow support for the head and raising the arm on the examination side is generally sufficient for small, non-pendulous breasts. The breast may be positioned in a way that it is stable and central on the chest wall by a small amount of rotation of the chest from a true supine position (**Figure 9.1**). This minimises the natural movement, which is inherent in the mature breast tissue of post-adolescent females. Large pendulous breasts will require lateral rotation of approximately 45° to access the lateral half of the breast. A semi-recumbent position may be required to image the upper half of the breast if it is overly large and so mobile that it falls towards the patient's face when supine.

Breast ultrasound employs a linear array transducer of high frequency, usually 7–10 MHz, sometimes as high as 14 MHz.[7]

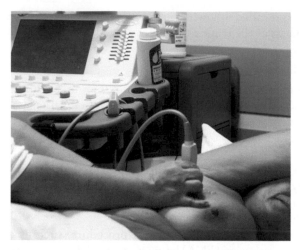

Figure 9.1 Positioning for breast sonography.

The breast may be examined by either target scanning, which is focusing on a specific area of interest, or whole breast examination. Target scans may be used in symptomatic clinics to examine the symptomatic quadrant and, if a suspicious mass is identified, then the whole of the breast and axilla are scanned. Sometimes the contralateral breast is also examined.

Documentation for mapping and reporting masses within the breast is usually performed using an imaginary clock face to represent the breast. The nipple is the centre of the clock and masses are located on the clock dial with a distance measured from the nipple in centimetres. The American College of Radiology (ACR) have standardised reporting guidance Breast Imaging – Reporting and Data System (BI-RADS).[8]

The method by which the breast quadrant is examined is dependent on the preference of the operator. Scanning techniques include transverse and longitudinal imaging within each quadrant of the clock, or radial scanning of the clock face around the nipple. Angulation of the transducer is essential to image the tissue posterior to the nipple as heavy shadowing from the nipple usually occurs. Lesions should be measured in at least two orthogonal planes and relevant images recorded.

Image analysis

The normal breast ultrasound appearances are of heterogeneous, hyperechoic glandular tissue, seen beneath hypoechoic fatty tissue (**Figure 9.2**).

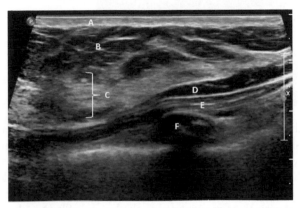

Figure 9.2 Sonogram of a normal breast. A. Dermis: note the half-centimetre scale along the right of the image, showing that this is about 2 mm in thickness. B. Superficial pre-mammary fat layer. C. Mammary layer; the glandular tissue of the breast. D. Retro-mammary fat layer. E. Pectoralis muscle. F. Rib: note the black acoustic shadowing beneath the rib surface.

A breast cyst (**Figure 9.3**) will usually have smooth, well-defined walls surrounding a rounded anechoic area with posterior acoustic enhancement. Occasionally there may be internal echoes, described as a complicated cyst.[8] Cysts may be single, multiple or septated. Galactoceles are cysts containing milk caused by a blocked lactiferous duct and usually appear as well-defined cysts, often with internal fluid levels. The fat content of the milk gives rise to a brighter appearance of the internal contents in some cases.

Abscesses are fluid filled and may contain some internal echoes, sometimes even gas. They have a thick, irregular border and usually occur around the nipple, although they may also be found at the periphery of the breast.

Fibroadenomas are usually ovoid, homogeneous in echotexture, with a regular border. They are often mobile when compressed.

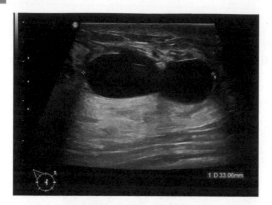

Figure 9.3 This image demonstrates two well-defined anechoic (no internal echoes) lesions characteristic of simple cysts.

Medullary carcinomas have a similar appearance to fibroadenomas, but are slightly more hyperechoic, with a well-defined border.

Invasive ductal carcinomas have an irregular border and homogeneous echotexture, with posterior attenuation (acoustic shadowing) in most cases (**Figure 9.4**). The irregular shape is a typical feature of the haphazard growth of malignancy as the lesion infiltrates the surrounding tissues. The mass is also poorly defined and is hypoechoic compared with the surrounding normal tissue. Thickening and indentation of the skin over the mass may also be seen.

Doppler assessment of vascularity of a breast mass may be helpful in differentiating benign from malignant lesions. Power Doppler is sensitive for detecting the low-volume blood flow typical of vascularising tumours (**Figure 9.5**).

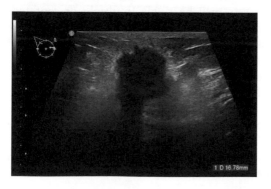

Figure 9.4 Irregularly shaped mass.

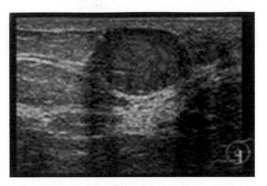

Figure 9.5 Power Doppler image of a breast mass.

CEUS is another useful adjunct for differentiation of suspicious lesions. It enables the assessment of the degree and pattern of vascularity within and around a lesion, including the presence of perfusion defects, and may better demonstrate the outline and homogeneity of a lesion. It is more sensitive than power Doppler in the evaluation of the microcirculation.[9]

ELASTOGRAPHY

Elastography, sometimes referred to as SonoElastography, is an electronically enhanced technique whereby a colour overlay relates to the stiffness of the tissue while scanning. The loss of elasticity in tissue is associated with tumour development or inflammatory conditions that lead to hardening of tissue, and the idea of breast palpation has long been based on this tissue property.

Elastography seeks to recognise these differences and demonstrate them by use of a colour overlay on the conventional B mode image. There are two types of elastography: (1) compression (or strain) elastography and (2) shear wave elastography (SWE).[10]

Compression elastography uses light compression by the operator during scanning. As gentle pressure is applied to the scanned area, the compressibility or elasticity of the tissue is calculated and compared between successive frames to compile a 'strain' map of comparative elasticity.

SWE uses special pulses within the ultrasound signal that can enable detection of tiny changes in the speed of sound due to changes in tissue stiffness. From these subtle changes, a quantitative value of the stiffness can be obtained. The relationship between a lesion and the surrounding normal tissue can also be expressed as a numerical value in terms of a strain ratio between the lesion and surrounding fatty tissue; ratios are calculated by dividing the mean strain within the lesion by the mean strain within the normal tissue.

Elastography can demonstrate some previously undetectable lesions and will show barely visible lesions more easily with a higher degree of accuracy than standard B mode imaging, improving the clinical diagnostic capability of breast sonography.[11]

Image analysis

The accompanying images demonstrate comparison of SWE with the greyscale (B mode) ultrasound. The scale is set to show more compressible or elastic structures in blue (**Figure 9.6**) and more rigid tissue structures in green or red (**Figure 9.7**).

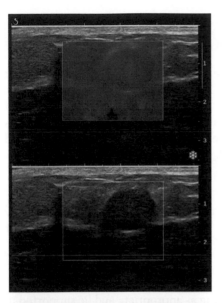

Figure 9.6 An elastography image (top) compared with the greyscale sonogram of a fibroadenoma in the breast. The colour overlay is uniformly blue, which according to the colour-coding scale (not shown on these images) indicates a softness of the lesion comparable with the surrounding tissue. Other visual appearances – ovoid shape, homogeneous echotexture and a regular border – in conjunction with the elastography image lead to a diagnosis of a fibroadenoma.

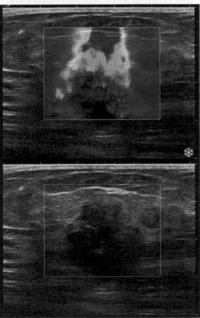

Figure 9.7 An elastography image (top) compared with the greyscale sonogram of a breast cancer. The lesion has a distinctly, differently coloured centre. The deep red zone in particular, being at the opposite end of the colour-coding scale, suggests a very stiff lesion. The B mode image is shown below the colour-coded elasticity map. It is heterogeneous, irregular and taller than it is wide. B mode and elastography together are suggestive of cancer.

VOLUME SCANNING

Volume scanning, or whole breast ultrasound (WBUS), is a breast ultrasound technique using a motor-driven wide transducer that traverses the skin surface over the breast. This allows acquisition of full-field volumes of the front, outer and inner sides of the breast.[12] It is also referred to as automated breast ultrasound (ABUS) or automated breast volume scanning (ABVS).

Indications

Volume scanning is used as an adjunct to mammography, especially for the denser breast, which is known to be a major risk factor for cancers.[13]

Patient preparation

The subject should remove clothing as appropriate and lie supported in the supine oblique position (**Figure 9.8**). The raised breast is covered with a single-use disposable mesh membrane, which aids breast stabilisation, compression, acoustic coupling and infection control.

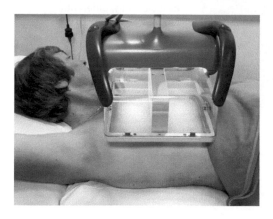

Figure 9.8 Whole breast ultrasound using an automated-motion transducer inside clear plastic housing.

Imaging procedure

A high-frequency (5–14 MHz) slightly concave probe, typically 15 cm in length, sits in a clear plastic paddle casing, which is lowered on to the breast. Some pressure is applied to compress the tissue and a pointer on the probe is aligned with the nipple.

A single pass is made to acquire transverse axial sections, followed by passes from a more lateral and then a more medial direction, to include the area extending longitudinally from the mid-axilla to the rib just beneath the breast, and transversely from the mid-sternum to the shoulder. Each pass takes approximately 40–60 seconds. More passes may be required to cover the larger breast. Each pass length is 17 cm, yielding a field view of 17 cm × 15 cm with a depth of 5–6 cm.

Image analysis

After image acquisition, a series of 2-mm coronal sections are reconstructed from the data and the operator marks the nipple location on the image; in **Figure** 9.9 the nipple marker is shown in blue. This image shows a normal ductal pattern. As with other three-dimensional (3D) digital imaging acquisition, further reconstructions enable visualisation in any desired plane.

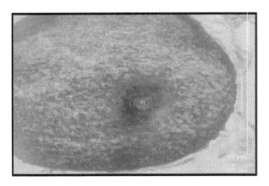

Figure 9.9 Reconstructed coronal section.

The images reconstructed in **Figure 9.10** demonstrate an invasive ductal carcinoma in the left breast of a 53-year-old woman. The carcinoma appears as a darker area, measuring 100 mm × 60 mm × 23 mm and best seen in the reconstructed coronal section.

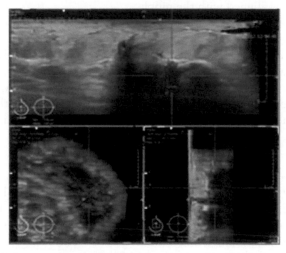

Figure 9.10 Reconstructed sections: transaxial (top), coronal plane (lower left) and sagittal (lower right).

The advantages of volume scanning are that it has decreased operator error on image acquisition[14] and enables greater coverage of breast tissue,[15] with whole lesions visible on single images for accurate measurement. Although reconstructions can be made at slice thicknesses as small as 0.5 mm, volume scanning is thought to have inferior image quality to conventional sonography, particularly around the subareolar region and in irregularly shaped and peripherally located lesions.[16] Technological developments to incorporate Doppler ultrasound and elastography with volume scanning may improve definition in the future.

REFERENCES

1. NICE (National Institute for Health and Care Excellence). *Early and locally advanced breast cancer: Diagnosis and treatment. Clinical guideline [CG80]*, 2017. Available at: https://www.nice.org.uk/Guidance/CG80.

2. Boyd NF, Guo H, Martin LJ, Sun L, Stone J, Fishell E, et al. Mammographic density and the risk and detection of breast cancer. *New England Journal of Medicine* 2007;**356**(3):227–236. doi: 10.1056/NEJMoa062790.

3. Folkman J. How is blood vessel growth regulated in normal and neoplastic tissue? G.H.A. Clowes memorial Award lecture. *Cancer Research* 1986;**46**(2):467–473. PMID: 2416426.

4. Advisory Committee on Breast Cancer Screening. *Screening for breast cancer in England: Past and future.* Journal of Medical Screening. 2006;**13**(2):59–61. doi: 10.1258/096914106777589678.

5. NICE (National Institute for Health and Care Excellence). *Familial breast cancer: Classification, care and managing breast cancer and related risks in people with a family history of breast cancer. Clinical guideline [CG164]*, 2019. Available at: https://www.nice.org.uk/Guidance/CG164.

6. UKHSA (UK Health Security Agency). Guidance. *Good infection prevention practice: Using ultrasound gel*, 2022. Available at: https://www.gov.uk/government/publications/ultrasound-gel-good-infection-prevention-practice/good-infection-prevention-practice-using-ultrasound-gel.

7. Szabo TL, Lewin PA. Ultrasound transducer selection in clinical imaging practice. *Journal of Ultrasound in Medicine* 2013;**32**(4):573–582. doi: 10.7863/jum.2013.32.4.573.

8. Mendelson EB, Böhm-Vélez M, Berg WA, Whitman GJ, Feldman MI, Madjar H, et al. *ACR BI-RADS Ultrasound.* In: D'Orsi CJ, Sickles EA, Mendelson EB, Morris EA (eds), *ACR BI-RADS Atlas: Breast Imaging Reporting and Data System*. Reston, VA: American College of Radiology, 2013:128–130. Available at: https://www.acr.org/Clinical-Resources/Reporting-and-Data-Systems/Bi-Rads#Ultrasound.

9. Boca Bene I, Dudea SM, Ciurea AI. Contrast-enhanced ultrasonography in the diagnosis and treatment modulation of breast cancer. *Journal of Personalized Medicine* 2021;**11**(2):81. doi: 10.3390/jpm11020081.

10. Barr RG. Sonographic breast elastography: A primer. *Journal of Ultrasound in Medicine* 2012;**31**(5):773–783. doi: 10.7863/jum.2012.31.5.773.

11. Gao LY, Gu Y, Xu W, Tian JW, Yin LX, Ran HT, et al. Can combined screening of ultrasound and elastography improve breast cancer identification compared with MRI in women with dense breasts – a multicenter prospective study. *Journal of Cancer* 2020;**11**(13):3903–3909. doi: 10.7150/jca.43326.

12. Wojcinski S, Farrokh A, Hille U, Wiskirchen J, Gyapong S, Soliman A, et al. The automated breast volume scanner (ABVS): Initial experiences in lesion detection compared with conventional handheld B-mode ultrasound: A pilot study of 50 cases. *International Journal of Women's Health* 2011;**3**:337–346. doi: 10.2147/IJWH.S23918.

13. Engmann NJ, Golmakani MK, Miglioretti DL, Sprague BL, Kerlikowske K; Breast Cancer Surveillance Consortium. Population-attributable risk proportion of clinical risk factors for breast cancer. *Journal of the American Medical Association Oncology* 2017;**3**(9):1228–1236. doi: 10.1001/jamaoncol.2016.6326.

14. Lin X, Wang J, Han F, Fu J, Li A. Analysis of eighty-one cases with breast lesions using automated breast volume scanner and comparison with handheld ultrasound. *European Journal of Radiology* 2012;**81**(5):873–878. doi: 10.1016/j.ejrad.2011.02.038.

15. Zhang Q, Hu B, Hu B, Li WB. Detection of breast lesions using an automated breast volume scanner system. *Journal of International Medical Research* 2012;**40**:300–306.

16. An YY, Kim SH, Kang BJ. The image quality and lesion characterization of breast using automated whole-breast ultrasound: A comparison with handheld ultrasound. *European Journal of Radiology* 2015;**84**(7):1232–1235. doi: 10.1016/j.ejrad.2015.04.007.

Further reading

Madjar H, Mendelson E. *The practice of breast ultrasound*, 2nd edn. Stuttgart: Thieme, 2008.

CHAPTER 10
THE CARDIOVASCULAR SYSTEM

The aorta   212
The extracranial arterial supply to the brain   217
Peripheral arterial – lower limb   223
Peripheral arterial – upper limb   230
Peripheral venous – lower limb   232
Peripheral venous – upper limb   237
Echocardiography   239
Transoesophageal echocardiography   249
Intravascular ultrasound   252
References   255

THE AORTA

Ultrasound is the ideal first-line imaging modality for examining the abdominal aorta because it is quick, relatively cheap and with no known side effects. The potential to use Doppler imaging to demonstrate movement makes this a particularly useful modality for imaging in the cardiovascular system. The thoracic aorta is less accessible and so ultrasonic imaging is generally restricted to the abdominal aorta.

The results of a randomised controlled trial, the Multicentre Aneurysm Screening Study,[1] demonstrated the potential to reduce mortality in men by the introduction of selective screening, and this has led to the introduction of UK-wide national screening programmes for abdominal aortic aneurysm (AAA), in addition to some local screening

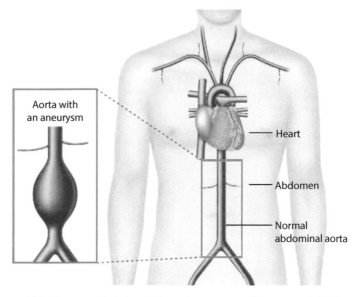

Figure 10.1 Diagram of abdominal aortic aneurysm (courtesy of the National Abdominal Aortic Aneurysm Screening Programme); the main picture shows a normal straight abdominal aorta, whereas the inset shows a bulge, characteristic of an aneurysm.

programmes. These utilise sonographic measurement of the aortic diameter to identify men at risk from rupture of an AAA (**Figure 10.1**). Screening is normally performed by specially trained technicians.

Indications

In the UK, men aged 65 are offered ultrasound screening for AAA under the National AAA Screening Programme (NAAASP). The national programme is restricted to men because they are six times more likely than women to die from a ruptured AAA.[1] Those with a family history of the condition may also benefit from screening and ultrasound screening offers a low-risk means of this.

Abdominal ultrasound is offered as an investigation for other high-risk patients, or those with clinical indications, for example a pulsatile mid-abdominal mass. It is used to monitor an identified aneurysm until it reaches the point where surgical intervention may occur and to assess the repair after surgery. Ultrasound is also useful for assessing associated conditions, for instance the renal arteries and the iliac arteries.

Immediately prior to AAA treatment, computed tomography (CT) imaging is performed to obtain precise dimensions for surgical planning, especially if a stent is required as these are tailored to fit the patient's specific anatomy. However, ultrasound is the preferred imaging modality for frequent use because of the relative speed, cost and radiation safety considerations.

Patient preparation

In the screening programme, there is no requirement for physical preparation, although subsequent scans are more successful after abdominal preparation of fasting or taking only clear fluids for several hours to reduce bowel gas that may affect image quality. As with any screening programme, there must be careful counselling to ensure that participants understand the risks, benefits and limitations of the procedure.

The abdomen is bared for ultrasound examination.

After the examination, the results may be conveyed to the patient in the case of the national screening programmes and/or to the referring clinician.

Imaging procedure

The patient lies supine on the couch and coupling gel is applied directly to the anterior abdominal wall. The abdomen is scanned using a 5.0 or 3.5 MHz curved array transducer in both longitudinal and transverse sections (**Figure 10.2**). Positive identification of the aorta is made by confirming the presence of the visible anterior branches, which are the coeliac axis and the superior mesenteric artery (**Figure 10.3**), and by checking that the other great vessel of the abdomen, the inferior vena cava (IVC), is compressible. In normal circumstances, the aorta should be non-compressible due to its strong arterial walls, and the IVC should be compressible provided that it is superficial enough to respond to the probe pressure and is not filled with thrombus or other pathology.

If an aneurysm is detected outside the screening programme, it is important to determine the level of the aneurysm in relation to the renal arteries. If the aneurysm is superior to the renal arteries the sonographer should check to see if there is a thoracic aneurysm. If this cannot be clearly identified, further imaging or a specialist opinion may be required.

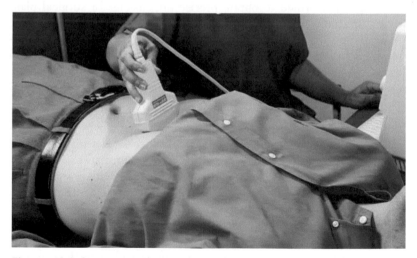

Figure 10.2 Scanning technique for abdominal aortic aneurysm screening: transverse section imaging. A paper towel is normally used to protect the clothing, but there is no need to undress, making the examination quicker and more acceptable to the patient.

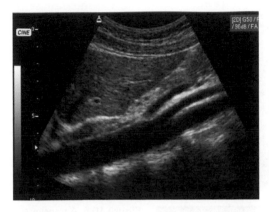

Figure 10.3 Sonogram of the normal aorta. Longitudinal section showing anterior branches – coeliac axis (more proximal) and superior mesenteric artery.

Image analysis

Greyscale ultrasound is usually sufficient to identify the aorta, particularly within screening programmes. Measurements are taken of the anteroposterior (AP) diameter in both longitudinal and transverse sections (**Figures 10.4** and **10.5**) and corrected to the nearest millimetre. The calibre of the aorta is considered to be within the normal range when it is up to 29 mm; an AP diameter of 30 mm and over is considered aneurysmal (**Figure 10.5**). Sometimes thrombus may be visible within the lumen of the aorta, usually appearing as more reflective, solid tissue (**Figure 10.6**).

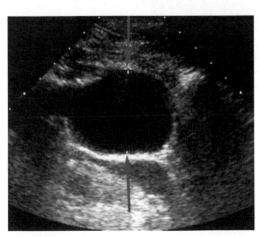

Figure 10.4 Sonogram of the normal aorta (courtesy of the National Abdominal Aortic Aneurysm Screening Programme); transverse section showing anteroposterior diameter measurement.

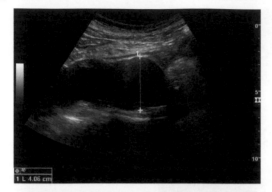

Figure 10.5 A longitudinal section of an aneurysmal aorta; this measurement would be corrected to 41 mm, which is aneurysmal. Note the tortuous path of the distended aorta.

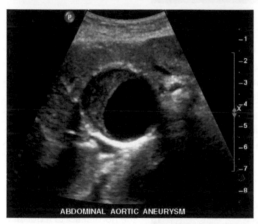

Figure 10.6 A transverse section of an aneurysmal aorta, with thrombus visible in the lumen.

In the pathological aorta, transverse or other measurements may be taken, and colourflow Doppler may be useful within the diagnostic scenario to demonstrate flow patterns where there is thrombus or dissection, and to check for endoleaks after surgery.

THE EXTRACRANIAL ARTERIAL SUPPLY TO THE BRAIN

The extracranial arterial supply to the brain comprises the carotid and vertebral arteries, which can be examined using ultrasound equipment with a combination of techniques. A good understanding of the vascular anatomy is required, including the many anatomical variants. Vessels can be demonstrated and blood flow assessed using real-time B mode imaging, spectral Doppler and colourflow Doppler. Ultrasound is the ideal imaging modality because it is quick and gives immediate and accurate measurements, as well as being excellent for investigating superficial structures and fluid-filled systems.

Indications

Ultrasound is useful in transient ischaemic attacks (TIAs) and stroke conditions, which may be associated with atherosclerotic lesions at the carotid bifurcation or neurological symptoms, which may be suggestive of subclavian steal syndrome or other symptoms suggestive of vascular disease. Carotid ultrasound is a recommended investigation for suspected stroke.[2,3]

Patient preparation

No particular preparation is required other than removing clothing and jewellery from around the neck region while ensuring patient comfort and privacy. Explanation of the sounds that will be audible when using Doppler can help patient expectations and understanding.

Imaging procedure

The patient is normally scanned in the supine position, with the neck extended and the head slightly turned away from the side being examined (**Figure 10.7**). Scanning from the cranial end of the couch may be ergonomically better for the sonographer, provided that there is sufficient arm support.

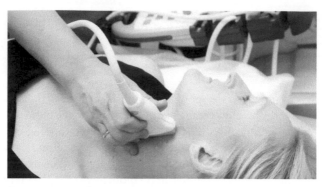

Figure 10.7 Positioning for scanning the carotid artery.

Using a 7–10 MHz linear array transducer, a transverse scan of the anterior vessels in the neck is performed immediately lateral to the thyroid gland, sweeping upwards and downwards to establish the course of the vessels. The position of the carotid bifurcation, where it divides into the external carotid artery (ECA) and internal carotid artery (ICA), is then located. The carotid arteries are also imaged in the longitudinal plane (**Figure 10.8**), and both sides are imaged for comparison.

Initial evaluation of the carotid arteries is by B mode imaging and, following identification and orientation, any plaque formation and its appearance are noted. Spectral Doppler is invaluable for quantitative assessment of flow in the carotid arteries, and the peak systolic and end-diastolic velocities are measured and recorded in the common carotid artery (CCA), ICA and ECA bilaterally.[4] Spectral Doppler measurements in the ECA tend to show pulsatile high-resistance, low diastolic flow, whereas in the ICA flow tends to be low resistance with a higher diastolic flow. Peak systolic velocities in the carotid arteries can vary depending on vessel size but are generally less than 120 cm/s in the normal ICA. The arteries each have slightly different flow characteristics, leading to an individual 'signature' audibly identifiable by the experienced operator using spectral Doppler.

The vertebral arteries may be imaged by angling the ultrasound beam slightly laterally from the CCA in long section. The vertebral artery should become visible between the vertebral processes of the cervical spine,[5] but this can be challenging in some cases and colour-flow Doppler imaging may be used as an adjunct to locate them.

Image analysis

The key to interpreting vascular imaging is to be sure of the orientation before starting to draw conclusions about direction of flow, because pathology may cause reversal of flow. The orientation of the images within this section is as per convention, with the cranial direction being to the left of the screen, but note that the colour scale varies because this is easily changed by means of the equipment controls, so this necessitates careful study in all colourflow Doppler images.

The B mode image in **Figure 10.8** shows a normal CCA at its bifurcation into the ECA, which is normally more medial at this level in the neck, and the ICA, which is therefore the more superficial vessel, although vascular anatomy is highly variable.

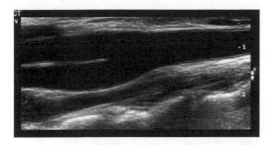

Figure 10.8 A longitudinal section of a normal common carotid artery, showing its bifurcation.

The colour scale in **Figure 10.9** shows that the red–yellow colours are flowing towards the probe and the blue colours away, and the slanting sides of the Doppler box shows that the receiving crystals are effectively more towards the left-hand side of the image as we are viewing it. Therefore, the moving blood in the carotid artery, which is the deeper structure, appears orange, showing that flow is coming towards the receiving crystals, or from right to left, and the blue colour in the more superficial jugular vein shows that flow is from left to right. As the probe orientation is correct, with the left side of the screen being towards the patient's head, this image shows that the flow in both vessels is in the correct direction.

Figure 10.10 depicts a normal carotid artery with smooth cephalad flow. This is a triplex image, comprising B mode with a colourflow Doppler overlay and the spectral Doppler waveform below. The spectral trace has a quantitative velocity scale, and the figures at the top right

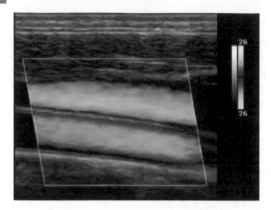

Figure 10.9 A duplex image (B mode and colourflow Doppler) of a normal common carotid artery and jugular vein; smooth flow is seen in both. Note the colour scale, which should always be included in Doppler images to facilitate interpretation.

of the image are the parameters for the systolic and diastolic speeds along with indicators of pulsatility and resistance derived from them. In this case, the peak systolic velocity (PSV or S) is 104 cm/s, which is well within the normal range. A high velocity would be diagnostic of a narrowing of the lumen, and the figures can be used to calculate the degree of stenosis with reasonable accuracy (**Figure 10.11**).

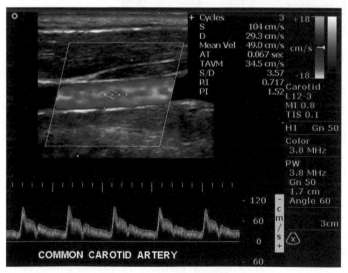

Figure 10.10 A triplex image: colourflow Doppler on the B mode image with spectral Doppler applied to measure the velocities.

Percentage stenosis (NASCET)	ICA PSV (cm/s)
<50	<125
50–69	>125
70–89	>230
>90	>400
Near occlusion	Trickle flow
Occlusion	No flow

Figure 10.11 A table showing the peak systolic velocity (PSV) of the internal carotid artery (ICA) and percentage stenosis, as shown in the North American Symptomatic Carotid Endarterectomy Trial (NASCET). (Table courtesy of Jain & Webb, 2012;[6] other tables are available.)

The colour scale indicates not only the direction of flow but also its speed; the highest velocities are represented by the palest colours, furthest away from the baseline, whereas the numbers at each end of the colour scale show the speed in centimetres per second at that colour. If the speed within the image exceeds the colour scale, it 'flips over' to the extreme end of the other half of the scale, an artefact known as aliasing.

Abnormal turbulent flow is shown in **Figure 10.12**, appearing as a mosaic of colours, with the palest shades representing the region of the highest velocities where aliasing has occurred. This is a stenotic lesion; a narrowing caused by plaque, in this case at the posterior aspect of the vessel, and characterised by an increase in blood velocity and often by turbulent flow in the vessel at that point and distal to the stenosis. A mix of colours may be indicative of either turbulence or the aliasing artefact. Both these conditions are demonstrated here; the darker colours just at the stenosis represent low-velocity turbulence, with blue being the back flow and the turquoise or light blue adjacent to the pale

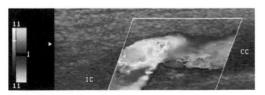

Figure 10.12 Colourflow Doppler of a stenosis at the carotid bifurcation. Turbulence and aliasing can be seen.

yellow is the high-velocity aliasing artefact. This is a useful indicator of the site of maximum velocity commonly distal to a stenosis, in this instance caused by atheromatous plaque at the bifurcation.

The sonographer can set the colour scale to use the aliasing artefact to best advantage in order to identify the site of maximum velocity within a vessel by colourflow Doppler. The scale is adjusted until aliasing occurs. Placing the spectral Doppler gate at this point allows the PSV to be measured for accurate estimation of the degree of stenosis in the vessel. Other calculations have been proposed,[7] but this method is in common usage.[4]

The vertebral arteries are similarly assessed using colourflow and spectral Doppler in order to determine whether there is anterograde flow, in other words the normal direction towards the head and brain, or abnormal retrograde flow away from the head. A vertebral artery is shown in **Figure 10.13**; the colour has been used in this instance to help identify the anatomy, which can be difficult to visualise.

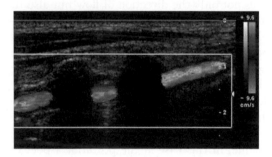

Figure 10.13 Duplex scan of the vertebral artery, visible as it passes between the cervical vertebrae.

The triplex image in **Figure 10.14** shows retrograde flow in the vertebral artery. This is indicative of subclavian steal syndrome, caused by blood pressure differentials and suggestive of severe stenosis or even occlusion in the subclavian artery proximal to the origin of the vertebral artery. Blood is 'stolen' from the vertebral artery to perfuse the arm, causing the retrograde flow.

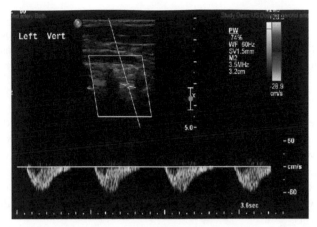

Figure 10.14 Retrograde flow in the vertebral artery in subclavian steal syndrome. Note that the spectral Doppler display is below the line, indicative of reversed flow in this case.

PERIPHERAL ARTERIAL – LOWER LIMB

Ultrasound is the ideal modality for the assessment of the location and extent of peripheral vascular disease because it is a relatively cost-effective, reproducible, painless and non-invasive modality. Vessels are examined using all types of pulsed wave imaging as well as continuous wave (CW) imaging, between which it is possible to perform detailed blood flow measurement and analysis. Sonography of the peripheral arterial system has shown results comparable with angiography.[8]

Indications

Investigations may be performed for assessment of congenital abnormalities, or for suspected narrowing and occlusion of vessels because of symptoms such as pains in the legs on exertion, ulcerations or discoloration of the extremities. Imaging may be performed following a poor ankle–brachial pressure index (ABPI), which itself is a sensitive measure of peripheral vascular disease, performed to determine the presence and extent of arteriopathy and to predict if there is sufficient perfusion to heal existing wounds and ulceration.[9]

Ultrasound diagnosis of occlusive arterial disease and assessment of the site and severity often take place before interventional procedures, such as angioplasty, and subsequently to assess the effectiveness of the procedure and to monitor the patency of a vascular graft or stent.

Patient preparation

The area to be examined must be bared, and this often includes parts proximal and distal to the affected area. Particularly when examining the lower limb, a covering should be offered to preserve privacy and dignity.

Infection control issues may need to be addressed more stringently when approaching intimate areas or, for example, in ulcerative conditions.

The ABPI

The ABPI is the ratio of the blood pressure in the legs to that in the arms, calculated by dividing the value of the highest systolic pressure at the ankle by the highest systolic blood pressure in the brachial artery of the arms.

Non-imaging CW Doppler ultrasound is used to obtain segmental pressure measurements at different locations along the limbs (**Figure 10.15**) to measure the systolic blood pressure values, which are used to

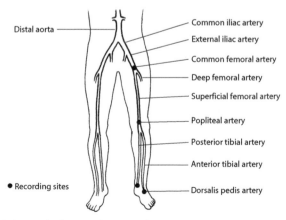

Figure 10.15 Lower limb recording sites for pressures.

calculate the ABPI. The small probe houses a dedicated CW transducer with a frequency of 8 MHz for the average ankle. A lower frequency (~5 MHz) may be used for an oedematous or otherwise enlarged limb.

The patient should be lying horizontally, so that the limbs to be measured are all at the same height. A sphygmomanometer cuff is inflated proximally to occlude arterial flow and released slowly to allow return of the flow. When a pulse is detected via the ultrasound probe, the systolic pressure is the same as the pressure in the cuff and is noted by the operator (**Figure 10.16**). The pressure in both arms should also be measured in case there is peripheral vascular disease in the upper

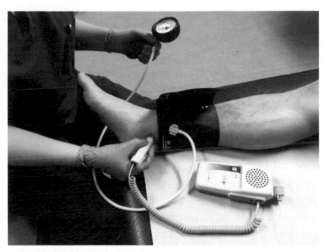

Figure 10.16 One of the measurements within the ankle–brachial pressure index examination.

limbs.[5] If the brachial pressures differ, the highest of these two readings should be used to calculate the ABPI.[10]

CW Doppler is used as an accurate measure of the systolic pressure because it is more sensitive than listening through a stethoscope, and the waveform patterns help in identifying normal or abnormal flow. Normally the ABPI is checked in the resting state, but sometimes the test is repeated after exercise.

The ABPI should be around 1.0, indicating a similar systolic pressure in the upper and lower limbs. A result below 0.9 or above 1.3 may indicate peripheral arterial disease and prompts the need for further investigations.

Note: there are no images for this procedure as it yields quantitative information only.

The operator in **Figure 10.16** is measuring the systolic blood pressure in the ankle, with the blood pressure cuff in position, and a CW Doppler probe and machine. Note that this machine does not have a screen and does not produce images. Instead, the operator listens to the audible Doppler signal to monitor the blood flow. The pressure readings are used to calculate the ABPI.

Imaging procedure

Ultrasound imaging of the lower limb arteries is performed with a linear array transducer of 3.5–7 MHz, using a combination of B mode, colourflow and spectral Doppler to assess the extent of any vascular disease in the limb. B mode imaging is used to follow the course of the vessel and visualise the presence of atherosclerotic disease.[11] Colourflow Doppler is used to demonstrate the blood flow, allowing identification of areas of stenosis, turbulence or occlusion. This allows accurate placement of the spectral Doppler sampling gate in the area of highest velocity, where spectral Doppler measures the maximum speed of blood flow through the narrowest points to enable calculation of the degree of stenosis in the vessel.

The patient is normally investigated supine with the legs spaced apart and the leg to be investigated externally rotated (**Figure 10.17**). The femoral artery is imaged here in the transverse plane to allow the operator to establish the course of the vessels and to locate the position of the femoral bifurcation. Imaging protocols may vary, but a common approach is then to scan the vessels with the probe in the longitudinal plane from the groin to the adductor canal in mid-thigh, with assessment of the common, deep and superficial femoral arteries (**Figure 10.18**).

The patient is then asked to turn on to their unaffected side to allow access to the popliteal fossa at the back of the knee of the affected leg. The probe is positioned to show the popliteal artery in the longitudinal plane, scanning down to the tibioperoneal trunk in the calf. In some cases, further imaging of the iliac and crural vessels may be performed.

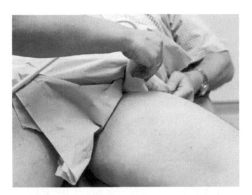

Figure 10.17 (left)
The patient's limb is externally rotated for a transverse scan of the common femoral artery, just proximal to its branching into the deep femoral artery and the superficial femoral artery.

Figure 10.18 (right)
The position for a longitudinal scan of the common femoral artery as it bifurcates into the superficial femoral artery and the deep femoral artery.

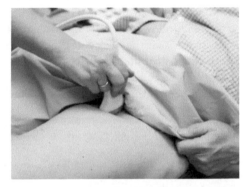

The vessels identified in transverse section (**Figure 10.19**) are examined in more detail in longitudinal sections. Any plaque formation and its appearance are noted on B mode. The dynamics of blood flow can be demonstrated using colourflow Doppler (**Figure 10.20**). Abnormal turbulent blood flow at a site may be demonstrated on the image as a mosaic of colours, the highest velocities normally being demonstrated as the palest shades.

A stenotic lesion, or narrowing caused by plaque in the vessel, is characterised by an increase in blood velocity and often by turbulent flow in the vessel within and distal to the stenosis. Spectral Doppler is invaluable for quantitative assessment of flow in the arteries, the waveform produced from each location provides information on any blood flow impairment and analysis can determine the area of stenosis and the extent of disease (**Figure 10.21**). The PSV is measured and recorded in the vessels examined and, although the pulsatility index may be calculated, it is less useful than the PSV at different points.[5] Some equipment may also facilitate measurement of the acceleration time, or rise time, which quantifies the rate at which the PSV is reached. Common femoral artery turbulence visible in the Doppler image, or a delayed rise time (>0.14 s), suggests iliac artery disease. Normally both limbs would be examined for comparison, as peripheral vascular disease is unlikely to be confined to one limb.[9]

Image analysis

The ultrasound image (**Figure 10.19**) is the starting point for a lower limb arterial examination. The common femoral artery (CFA) is identified and followed distally in this examination. It often appears, as on this image, as if the CFA and the common femoral vein (CFV) are one continuous fluid area, however this is an artefactual appearance due to lack of plane reflection from the sidewalls of vessels. The other vessel on the image is the long saphenous vein (LSV).

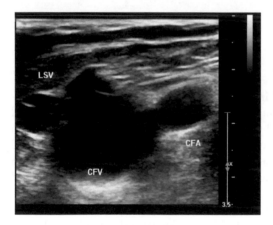

Figure 10.19 A normal transverse section of the vessels in the left groin, showing the common femoral artery (CFA), common femoral vein (CFV) and long saphenous vein (LSV).

A longitudinal section of the normal CFA is shown in **Figure 10.20** with colourflow Doppler. Assuming that the operator is holding the probe to comply with the positioning convention of having the patient's head to the left of the screen, the colour bar scale shows that flow is from left to right, because the slant of the colour box indicates that the receiving crystals are sited more to the right of the image. This means that flow is afferent, as it should be in an artery. The consistent red coloration indicates that flow is smooth, suggesting that this is a normal vessel; the exact interpretation should always be made by the sonographer at the time of examination, as this is highly dependent on equipment settings and relative motion and position of the operator and patient.

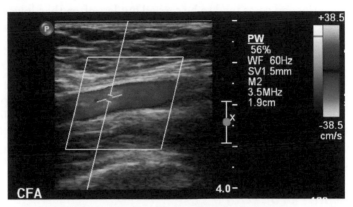

Figure 10.20 Duplex scan of the common femoral artery (CFA).

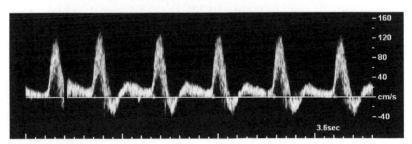

Figure 10.21 A normal spectral Doppler trace of the common femoral artery at the same point as **Figure 10.20**. This is a normal triphasic waveform, demonstrating good elasticity in the vessel walls.

PERIPHERAL ARTERIAL – UPPER LIMB

Although studies using B mode, colourflow and spectral Doppler may be undertaken to investigate arterial disease in a similar way to that described in the lower limbs, ultrasound examinations of the upper limb arteries and veins tend to be carried out less often than lower limb studies, because of the lower prevalence of atherosclerotic disease in the upper limb.[12]

Indications

The most common indication for ultrasound of the arterial supply to the upper limb is probably for suspected thoracic outlet syndrome (TOS) to distinguish between neurogenic and vascular causes of TOS. The subclavian artery should be scanned to check for compression by muscle hypertrophy or an accessory rib.

Imaging procedure

Using a linear array transducer with a frequency of 7–12 MHz and the patient initially supine (**Figure 10.22**), the subclavian, brachial, radial, ulnar and digital arteries may be assessed.

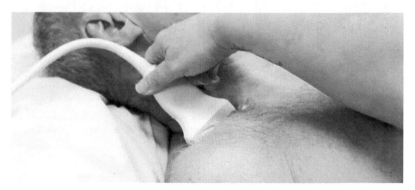

Figure 10.22 A patient positioned for an ultrasound examination of the subclavian artery, which is generally accessed supraclavicularly. It is important to evaluate flow in the symptomatic position,[8] so the position will be varied, as explained within the text.

When examining the subclavian artery, it is crucial to make a positive identification of the vessel using colourflow Doppler (**Figure 10.23**), as the subclavian vein is in close proximity and is highly pulsatile.[9]

Segmental systolic blood pressures of the more distal arteries can be measured using the method described in this chapter in the section on 'The ABPI'. Readings are taken with the arms in various positions to determine whether loss of signal is the result of compression of the subclavian artery; first with the patient standing or sitting with their arms by the side of the thorax; second with the shoulders held back and down and the head turned towards the affected side; and third with the arm hyperabducted at 90° and 180°.

Depending on symptoms, this examination may be undertaken in conjunction with ultrasound of the vertebral arteries to check for subclavian steal (see the section on 'The extracranial arterial supply to the brain' in this chapter).

Image analysis

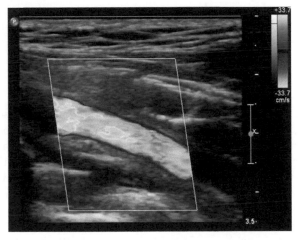

Figure 10.23 A duplex (B mode and colourflow Doppler) scan in longitudinal section of the distal subclavian artery with normal flow. Aliasing is seen as the palest blue in the middle of the vessel, indicating that this is where the peak velocities are. There is no visible compression of the artery within this section.

PERIPHERAL VENOUS – LOWER LIMB

Indications

- Assessment of varicose veins, to check their suitability for surgical intervention, and after the procedure to assess the success.
- Marking of veins for 'harvesting' as conduit grafts.
- Suspicion of deep venous thrombosis (DVT); presenting symptoms are commonly leg swelling and/or oedema.
- Location of arteriovenous malformations (AVMs) and other vascular anomalies.

Patient preparation

The patient must remove clothing from the area to be examined, which often includes the areas proximal and distal to the affected area. Care should be taken to maintain dignity, and a clean sheet or paper towel is normally used to cover the areas not being examined. Infection control is particularly important when scanning close to surgical scars, ulcerative or intimate areas.

Imaging procedure

The lower limb veins are examined with the patient in a reverse Trendelenburg position on a tilting examination couch, or in some cases standing. A 3.5–7 MHz linear array transducer is probably best suited to the range of depths encountered in the investigation of the veins of the lower limb. The probe is positioned against the skin over the area of the affected vein and a transverse scan is performed to locate the vessel. The vessel is also scanned in the longitudinal plane, with the transducer moved both distally and proximally along the length of the vessel.

Duplex imaging – real-time B mode imaging combined with colour-flow Doppler – is the preferred initial investigation for the diagnosis of DVT in the CFV, femoral and popliteal veins.[13] The probe is used to apply gentle pressure while observing in real time if the section of vein is readily compressed, which would indicate a normal vein, or if it retains its dimensions, which is indicative of the presence of a thrombus.

The additional use of colourflow Doppler may sometimes demonstrate blood flow around a thrombus in the partly occluded vessel.

Varicose veins are normally caused by incompetence in either the LSV, which runs medially from the ankle to the groin, or the short saphenous vein (SSV), which runs from the calf to the posterior aspect of the knee. When investigating for varicose veins, the patient may be asked to perform the Valsalva manoeuvre in order to demonstrate whether or not the valves within the veins are functioning properly by preventing reverse flow. More distally in the lower thigh and calf, augmentation is carried out by squeezing the calf, and checking for reverse flow immediately following augmentation. Augmentation acts in a similar way to the Valsalva manoeuvre to increase pressure and demonstrate venous insufficiency (previously known as incompetence), if present. Any reflux is an indication of valve insufficiency.

Colourflow and spectral Doppler can also be used in more detailed venous ultrasound examinations to diagnose the sites of incompetence and incompetent perforating veins, which cause varicose vein abnormalities. The vascular sonographer is able to give the clinician very detailed information about the course, diameter and tortuosity of the vessels, including how they connect with varicose veins. This information allows careful planning of treatment for the condition by the vascular surgeons.

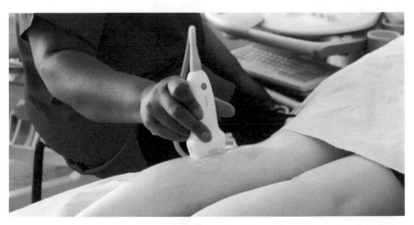

Figure 10.24 Position and technique for examination of the leg veins; this shows the probe position for the mid-calf veins in longitudinal section.

Image analysis

In varicose vein studies, incompetence may be shown within the deep or superficial veins. Highlighting this to the surgeon allows them to plan treatment options.

Figures 10.25 and **10.26** show a transverse section of the calf, with the probe rotated through 90° from the position shown in **Figure 10.24**. The Duplex image in **Figure 10.26** has a colourflow Doppler overlay, showing there is flow through the vein and, therefore, it is patent and with a competent proximal valve. Without the aid of a Doppler, it is not always possible to tell if the vessel is patent; if it is occluded by fresh thrombus the greyscale appearance is very similar, but there would be no colourflow signal. Often, the patient is imaged standing, particularly to check for varicose veins, as the effect of gravity helps to show this.

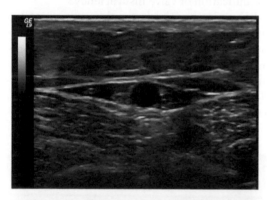

Figure 10.25 The short saphenous vein (SSV) in the calf; the probe is at a similar level to **Figure 10.24**, although this is a transverse section.

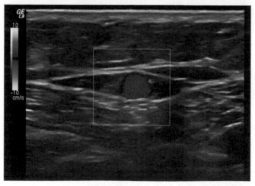

Figure 10.26 A duplex image in the same section as **Figure 10.25**.

A *triplex* scan uses three modes: greyscale, colourflow Doppler and spectral Doppler as seen in **Figure 10.27**. It demonstrates flow through the CFV, and the spectral Doppler trace is of normal phasic flow for a vein; compare this with the much more pulsatile spectral Doppler traces of the arteries and the heart.

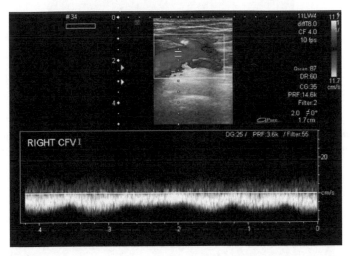

Figure 10.27 A triplex image at the level of the groin, showing the common femoral vein (CFV).

The right saphenofemoral junction (SFJ) should be scanned in the transverse section (**Figure 10.28**), to demonstrate where the LSV meets the CFV. Immediately lateral to the SFJ the CFA can be seen. The three vessels are often thought of as a 'Mickey Mouse' view, with the CFV being the head and the CFA and the LSV being the ears. When compression is applied at the SFJ, the LSV is easily compressed, losing one of the 'ears' of the Mickey Mouse view (**Figure 10.29**). If thrombus were present, the vein would remain patent.

The two methods of assessing for the presence of thrombus (its compressibility and the assessment of the haemodynamics by Doppler ultrasound) are both used in a thorough examination to increase the confidence of the results.

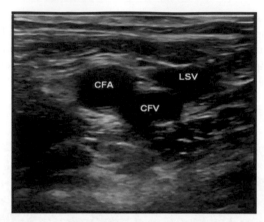

Figure 10.28 A transverse section at the level of the right groin, showing the right sapheno-femoral junction in transverse section. CFA, common femoral artery; CFV, common femoral vein; LSV, long saphenous vein.

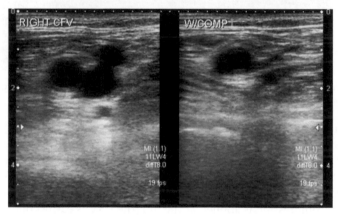

Figure 10.29 The saphenofemoral junction, uncompressed (left) and with compression (right). CFV, common femoral vein.

PERIPHERAL VENOUS – UPPER LIMB

The upper limb veins may be scanned using similar techniques to those employed for the lower limb. The internal jugular, subclavian, axillary and brachial veins can be checked for compressibility and flow, using a combination of B mode and colourflow Doppler.

Indications

Repeated catheter access or intravenous drug abuse may cause damage such as phlebitis or DVT. A suspected DVT is the main pathology affecting the venous system in the upper limb, and this is the most common indication for ultrasound investigations.[5] The upper limb is not a common site for varicose veins.

Imaging procedure

The patient should lie supine with the arm abducted and supported. A linear array transducer with a frequency of 7–12 MHz is used to obtain images in the longitudinal and transverse sections of each vein under consideration. The more distal and especially the more superficial veins should appear compressible on B mode scanning if they are normal; a DVT will generally be non-compressible unless it is very fresh thrombus.

Flow within the subclavian vein can be assessed using the Valsalva manoeuvre, which should cause a reverse- or no-flow state, followed by a surge towards the heart during exhalation.

Image analysis

When a DVT is present B mode ultrasound can show mixed internal echoes within the lumen of the vessel, which should normally appear echo free. In **Figure 10.30**, the brachial vein appears to be completely filled with thrombus.

Less dense thrombus in the left axillary vein is demonstrated in **Figure 10.31**. Here, colourflow Doppler has been used to try to pick up any movement, and a small red area visible in the lower right quadrant of the colour box is the only flow. Power Doppler is more sensitive to low-flow states and might demonstrate the extent of any remaining patency in such a situation. **Figure 10.32** is a transverse section across the same area, and occlusion is seen as a grey area (labelled OCC) where there should be a visible lumen.

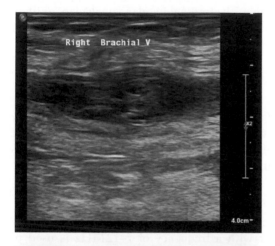

Figure 10.30 The right brachial vein (V).

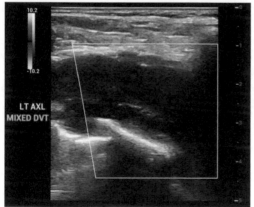

Figure 10.31 Duplex image: B mode and colourflow Doppler sonogram of the left (LT) axillary (AXL) vein. DVT, deep vein thrombosis.

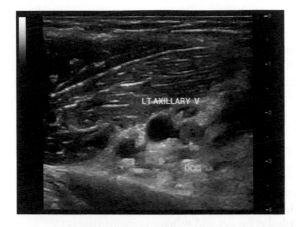

Figure 10.32 The left axillary vein (V) in transverse section in the same patient. The green label OCC marks the area of occlusion.

ECHOCARDIOGRAPHY

Cardiac ultrasound, otherwise known as echocardiography, offers a non-invasive method of examining the heart using two-dimensional (2D) real-time ultrasound, including M mode and Doppler. Both qualitative and quantitative information relating to heart disease and function are readily obtainable and, in many cases, echocardiography is the only imaging modality selected. The investigation is accomplished with specialised ultrasound equipment using a small footprint, phased array probe, usually with a transducer frequency range of 4–7 MHz. Two-dimensional B mode imaging is employed initially, and then used to direct M mode and Doppler studies. Information from the different studies can be displayed on the same monitor in either dynamic or still images, along with a record of an electrocardiogram (ECG) tracing if this is taken during the examination. As well as anatomical information, this enables evaluation of various features such as flow velocities and volumes, and both still images and real-time clips can be recorded to give a permanent record of the procedure that can be reviewed and used to assess changes in the cardiac condition.

As compared with the other main modalities in cardiac imaging (nuclear cardiology, cardiac MRI and cardiac CT), echocardiography is the cheapest, most mobile and most readily available; it avoids the disadvantage of using ionising radiation, and has no contraindications due to claustrophobia, renal failure or implanted devices. It gives superior assessment of diastolic and valvular function and can be used in conjunction with physiological or pharmacological stress testing.[14]

Indications (for both transthoracic and transoesophageal examinations)

Conditions such as arrhythmia or breathlessness may suggest investigations for congenital heart disease, myocardial abnormalities, tumours, valve disease, pericardial effusion and ischaemic heart disease.

Patient preparation

The patient is usually supported in a supine or semi-recumbent position to enable access to the chest while avoiding any breathing difficulties that may arise in some patients if they lie completely flat. The chest is bared and a small amount of coupling gel applied to the appropriate access points. In this position, the heart is examined in the long and short axes in order to assess its anatomy and function.

The patient is rotated approximately 50° towards the left side for further long axis, short axis, apical four chamber and 'five chamber' views. This rotation allows the heart to assume a position closer to the chest wall to enable better imaging.

Imaging procedure

A typical imaging protocol comprises five sections of the heart, starting with the parasternal long axis section and continuing with the short axis, apical four chamber, five chamber and subcostal sections. The ultrasound probe is positioned at selected locations for each section, as shown in **Figures 10.33–10.37** and explained in **Figure 10.38**.

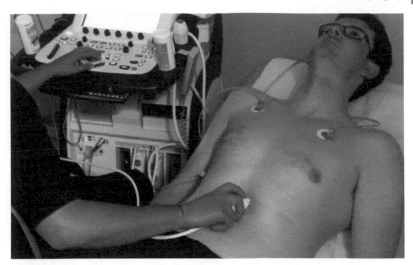

Figure 10.33 Patient lying semi-recumbent, the initial position for an 'echo' examination. This shows the subcostal approach.

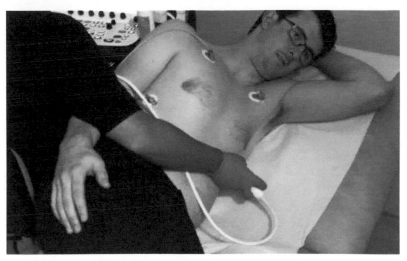

Figure 10.34 Patient rotated to the left to allow closer access from the chest wall to the heart. The probe is directed towards the apex of the heart.

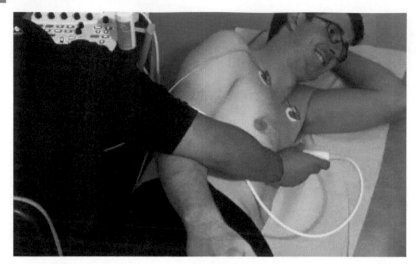

Figure 10.35 The patient is still rotated to the left, but this time the probe is held in the parasternal position to obtain different cross-sections of the heart.

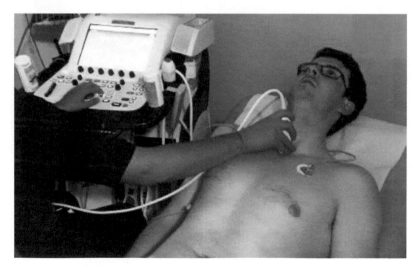

Figure 10.36 With the patient semi-recumbent, the suprasternal approach will demonstrate the aortic arch and descending aorta.

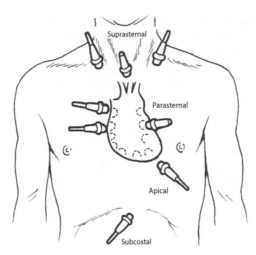

Figure 10.37 Different probe positions to obtain the standard sections.

Probe position	Section
In the suprasternal notch	Suprasternal section
In the left fourth intercostal notch	Long axis parasternal Short axis parasternal
From below the cardiac apex	Apical four chamber Apical five chamber
From under the xiphoid cartilage	Subcostal section

Figure 10.38 The sections obtained with the various probe positions in **Figure 10.37**

These probe locations represent acoustic windows, avoiding air in the lungs and bony structures such as the ribs and sternum. Careful angulation of the probe from these locations will facilitate visualisation of different anatomical details at oblique angles from the planes selected. Real-time scanning enables observation of cardiac wall motion and valve function. Cardiac dimensions can also be measured from static images, enabling calculation of valve area cross-sections and ventricular size.

The dynamics of blood flow can be visualised using colourflow Doppler. Although this is useful in many areas of heart disease, it is particularly helpful in congenital problems, for instance in visualising septal defects.

M mode studies are performed in conjunction with 2D echocardiography to assess function of the left ventricle, aortic valve and mitral valve. During acquisition, ECG tracings may be recorded simultaneously to enable accurate timing of events in the cardiac cycle. M mode is best selected in the long and short axis views to produce tracings of the movement of cardiac anatomy perpendicular to the ultrasonic beam. M mode has excellent temporal resolution and is a good complementary technique to Doppler studies.[15]

Spectral, colourflow and CW Doppler enable evaluation of blood flow patterns and velocities through the heart chambers and valves. To ensure accurate velocity measurements, the probe should be positioned to align the beam as closely as possible with the direction of blood flow.

The efficiency of the heart valves can be assessed by positioning the sample volume cursor at the site of the valve and studying the velocity, direction of flow, timing and intensity of the spectral information obtained. Jets of blood associated with stenotic valves can be observed, as well as the regurgitation of blood associated with incompetent valves. This can be seen with either colourflow Doppler or pulsed wave spectral Doppler. However, this detects only a limited range of the flow velocities possible within the heart; if the peak velocity exceeds this range, aliasing artefact occurs, rendering measurements inaccurate. CW Doppler overcomes this problem, as it can measure much higher velocities, but it has the disadvantage that the location of the sample along the line of interrogation cannot be pinpointed.

Image analysis

The duplex image of **Figure 10.39** shows both B mode and colourflow Doppler in a long axis section of the heart. The right ventricle is nearest to the probe, with the left ventricle beyond, and the aortic root is to the right of the image. The Doppler scale indicates blood flow away from the operator through the aortic valve (blue) and towards the operator (red) in the left atrium. This is the normal configuration and pattern of flow.

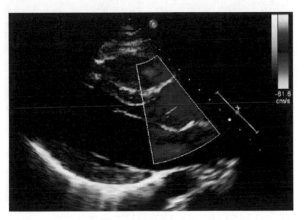

Figure 10.39 A long axis view from the parasternal approach.

The short axis view (**Figure 10.40**) shows the aortic valve in the centre of the image. The right ventricle is nearer to the probe, with the right atrium at the lower left part of the image and the left atrium in the low centre.

The M mode tracing in **Figure 10.41** shows the right ventricular motion and the excursion of the anterior and posterior mitral valve leaflets. From these tracings, various parameters may be measured and calculated: ventricular wall thickness, chamber size, contractility and ejection fraction. Valve thickness is determined and the degree of valve movement assessed along with the rate of valve opening and closing, and the information is used to estimate the severity of any valve stenosis.

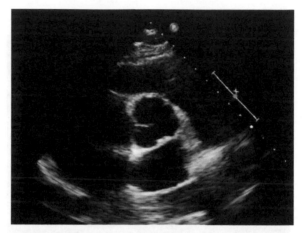

Figure 10.40 Short axis view at the level of the aortic valve.

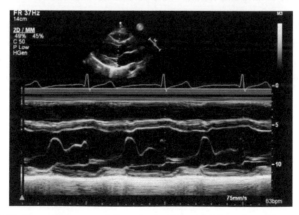

Figure 10.41 B mode image of the mitral valve with M mode tracing.

The diagram in **Figure 10.42** shows the structures of the heart as the beam passes through them from different angles via a parasternal approach, with a key to these structures beneath. These three sections will produce three different M mode traces, as depicted by the three diagrams on the right.

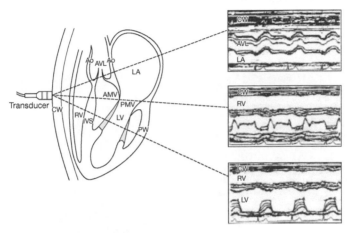

Figure 10.42 Three sections through the heart with their M mode tracings. AMV, anterior mitral valve leaflets; Ao, aorta; AVL, aortic valve leaflets; CW, chest wall; IVS, interventricular septum; LA, left atrium; LV, left ventricle; PMV, posterior mitral valve leaflets; PW, posterior LV wall; RV, right ventricle.

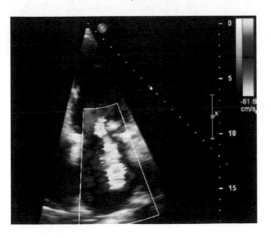

Figure 10.43 Duplex image of the mitral valve.

The different colours of the Doppler signal in **Figure 10.43** relate to the velocities at each point, as indicated by the colour scale on the right of the image. The overall picture is one of some backflows with turbulence, indicating moderate mitral valve regurgitation.

The upper part of **Figure 10.44** uses a colourflow Doppler overlay on the B mode image of the heart to allow positioning through the mitral valve, with the 'line of sight' of the spectral Doppler tracing in the lower part of the image. The Doppler trace gives peak velocity measurements and demonstrates moderate regurgitation of the mitral valve.

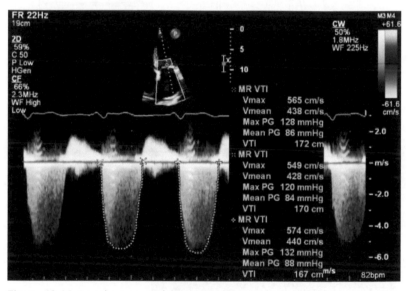

Figure 10.44 A triplex image of the mitral valve.

TRANSOESOPHAGEAL ECHOCARDIOGRAPHY

Patient preparation

Patients undergoing TOE are starved for 4 hours prior to the procedure, which is performed under light sedation.

Imaging procedure

Transoesophageal echocardiography (TOE) is performed using a 5 to 8 MHz transoesophageal probe. The tiny probe is introduced using an endoscope, while the patient is under light sedation. The transoesophageal probe is shown in **Figure 10.45**; the actual transducer is the area at the tip of the black tubing, which is inserted orally. There are controls on the shaft to direct the transducer once in situ.

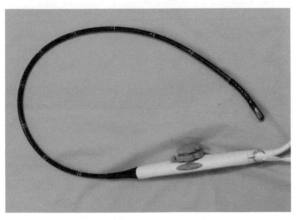

Figure 10.45 A transoesophageal cardiac probe.

This technique gives better image detail, particularly of the atria and the valves, because the probe is so much closer to the heart than with standard transthoracic echocardiography. If the left ventricular function needs to be evaluated, the probe is advanced into the stomach for a transgastric view. This can also demonstrate any pericardial effusions quite effectively. Although this procedure will produce much more detailed images, it does carry all the risks of endoscopy.[16]

Image analysis

The images shown are standard sections in keeping with the British Society of Echocardiography protocol.[17]

The right ventricular inflow and outflow at the level of the mid-oesophagus are shown in **Figure 10.46**, enabling evaluation of right ventricular function. In this image, the three leaflets of the tricuspid valve are clearly seen.

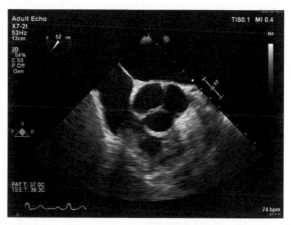

Figure 10.46 A section from the mid-oesophageal region, with 60–80° of rotation

A split-screen image, also from the mid-oesophageal area, showing the long axis of the heart is shown in **Figure 10.47**, enabling assessment of left ventricular function. The outflow tract from the left ventricle can be seen as the echo-free area in the left image. The right image, with a colourflow Doppler overlay, shows that there is some aortic regurgitation and turbulence at the valve.

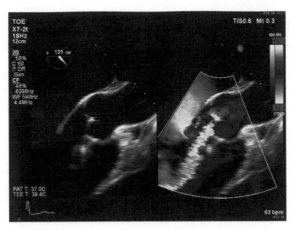

Figure 10.47 Long axis views; 20–150° of rotation.

The 3D reconstruction in **Figure 10.48** shows a replacement mechanical mitral valve.

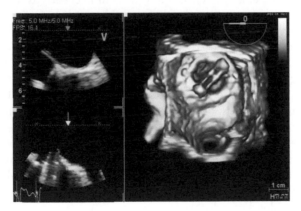

Figure 10.48 Three-dimensional reconstruction images.

INTRAVASCULAR ULTRASOUND

Intravascular ultrasound (IVUS) is a technique for examining the inside of a blood vessel using a tiny ultrasound transducer that is passed through the lumen of a vessel, often as part of minimally invasive heart surgery.

This plays an important role before and during interventional procedures in providing information on the type and extent of disease, enabling the clinician to select the most appropriate interventional procedure. Unlike optical coherence tomography (OCT), which can also be performed during angiography, IVUS enables visualisation of the structures beyond the lumen and the visible wall of the vessel.

Indications

- IVUS is performed during cardiac angiography and more particularly during angioplasty, when it is often necessary to examine the lumen of the artery to a level of detail beyond the capability of the coronary angiogram and depth unachievable with OCT. It can be used to measure the true diameter of an artery across the tunica intima. This will assist in the selection of the optimal balloon size for angioplasty.
- IVUS can demonstrate atheroma or plaque distribution, thickness and composition. This yields qualitative information, enabling characterisation of tissue pathology, so that it is possible to differentiate lesions that are fibrotic, lipidic (fatty), necrotic or calcified. This enables the cardiologist to select appropriate techniques such as thrombectomy or rotablation. It is also possible to calculate the percentage stenosis within a vessel, and of course this is applicable to other blood vessels.[18]
- IVUS assists in the management of stenting and atherectomy and is a particularly useful adjunct to coronary arteriography in bifurcation stenting, ostial lesions, long segments and left main stenting.[19]
- After stenting, IVUS can evaluate the lumen and check that the stent is firmly and closely apposed to the tunica media of the coronary artery. If this is not the case, there is a high likelihood that

the stenosis will reoccur within the stent. This is termed in-stent re-stenosis.

Patient preparation

IVUS is a technique performed during angiography. There is no additional preparation necessary.

Imaging procedure

Once angiography has located a stenosis in the selected coronary vessel, a guidewire is passed beyond the stenosis. A special IVUS catheter is passed using the conventional over-the-guidewire technique to facilitate introduction of the ultrasound endoprobe. Older equipment may use a motor drive unit to power a rotating mechanical sector scanner of 10–30 MHz, but more modern technology employs an electronic annular array transducer capable of frequencies of up to 40 MHz. The former produces a sector-shaped image, whereas the latter can produce a complete circular image, provided that there is no interruption in the field of view by the presence of other equipment.[20] Both systems produce real-time cross-sectional imaging of the endoluminal structures of the coronary arteries, enabling the structure of the arterial walls to be interrogated, as well as any existent plaque.

Image analysis

These images are produced by an electronic annular array transducer, giving 360° field of view. **Figure 10.49** is an axial view of a normal vessel, the black void in the centre being the probe itself.

Figure 10.50 shows an atherosclerotic vessel, which has some atheromatous deposits with calcification in the tunica intima. The yellow outlined area shows the true lumen of the vessel, the calcification is outlined in blue and the large arc outlined in orange beyond this is an acoustic shadow characteristic of these findings.

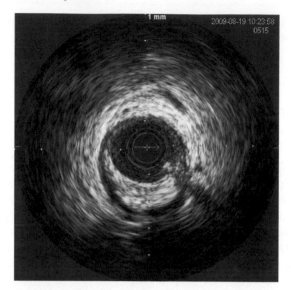

Figure 10.49 A normal coronary artery.

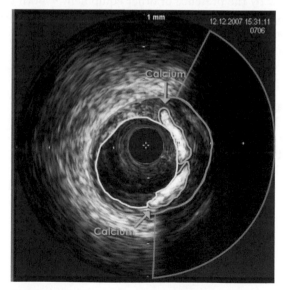

Figure 10.50 Typical features of an atherosclerotic artery.

REFERENCES

1. Ashton HA, Buxton MJ, Day NE, Kim LG, Marteau TM, Scott RA, et al. The Multicentre Aneurysm Screening Study (MASS) into the effect of abdominal aortic aneurysm screening on mortality in men: A randomised controlled trial. *The Lancet* 2002;**360**(9345):1531–1539. doi: 10.1016/s0140-6736(02)11522-4.

2. Ricotta JJ, AbuRahma A, Ascher E, Eskandari M, Faries P, Brajesh K. Updated Society for Vascular Surgery guidelines for management of extracranial carotid disease. *Journal of Vascular Surgery* 2011;**54**(3):e1–e31. doi: 10.1016/j.jvs.2011.07.031.

3. Bowen A, James M, Young G. (eds.). *National clinical guideline for stroke*, 5th edn. London: Royal College of Physicians of London, 2016.

4. Oates CP, Naylor AR, Hartshorne T, Charles SM, Fail T, Humphries K, et al. Joint recommendations for reporting carotid ultrasound investigations in the United Kingdom. *European Journal of Vascular and Endovascular Surgery* 2009;**37**(3):251–261. doi: 10.1016/j.ejvs.2008.10.015.

5. Thrush A, Hartshorne T. *Vascular ultrasound: How, why and when.* London, Churchill Livingstone, 2010.

6. Jain A, Webb J. A beginner's guide to grading of carotid artery stenosis by doppler ultrasound, CT and MR angiography – A correlative multimodality approach. *European Congress of Radiology* 2012. Poster C-2335. doi: 10.1594/ecr2012/C-2335.

7. Hathout GM, Fink JR, El-Saden SM, Grant EG. Sonographic NASCET index: A new doppler parameter for assessment of internal carotid artery stenosis. *American Journal of Neuroradiology* 2005;**26**(1):68–75. PMID: 15661704.

8. Pemberton M, London NJ. Color flow duplex imaging of occlusive arterial disease of the lower limb. *British Journal of Surgery* 1997;**84**(7):912–919. doi: 10.1002/bjs.1800840706.

9. Daigle RJ. *Techniques in non-invasive vascular diagnosis*, 4th edn. Littleton, CO: Summer Publishing, 2014.

10. Ruff D. Doppler assessment: Calculating an ankle brachial pressure index. *Nursing Times* 2003;**99**(42):62–65. PMID: 14618994.

11. Craiem D, Chironi G, Graf S, Denarié N, Armentano RL, Simon A. Atheromatous plaque: Quantitative analysis of the echogenicity of different layers. *Revista Española de Cardiologia* 2009;**62**(9):984–991. doi: 10.1016/S1885-5857(09)73264-5.

12. Abou-Zamzam AM Jr, Edwards JM, Porter JM. Non-invasive diagnosis of upper extremity disease. In: AbuRahma AF, Bergan JJ (eds), *Non-invasive vascular diagnosis*. London: Springer, 2000:269.
13. Beyer J, Schellong S. Deep vein thrombosis: Current diagnostic strategy. *European Journal of Internal Medicine* 2005;**16**(4):238–246. doi: 10.1016/j.ejim.2005.04.001.
14. Shah BN. Echocardiography in the era of multimodality cardiovascular imaging. *BioMed Research International* 2013;2013:310483. doi: 10.1155/2013/310483.
15. Feigenbaum H. Role of M-mode technique in today's echocardiography. *Journal of the American Society of Echocardiography* 2010;**23**(3):240–257; 335–357. doi: 10.1016/j.echo.2010.01.015.
16. Flachskampf FA, Badano L, Daniel WG, Feneck RO, Fox KF, Fraser AG, et al. Recommendations for transoesophageal echocardiography: Update 2010. *European Journal of Echocardiography* 2010;**11**(7):557–576. doi:10.1093/ejechocard/jeq057.
17. Wheeler R, Steeds R, Rana B, Wharton G, Smith N, Allen J, et al. A minimum dataset for a standard transoesophageal echocardiogram: A guideline protocol from the British Society of Echocardiography. *Echo Research and Practice* 2015;**2**(4):G29–G45. doi: 10.1530/ERP-15-0024.
18. Diethrich EB, Irshad K, Reid DB. Virtual histology and color flow intra-vascular ultrasound in peripheral interventions. *Seminars in Vascular Surgery* 2006;**19**(3):155–162. doi: 10.1053/j.semvascsurg.2006.06.001.
19. Tyczyński P, Chmielak Z, Pręgowski J, Rewicki M, Karcz M. Intervention on the left main coronary artery. Importance of periprocedural and follow-up intra-vascular ultrasonography guidance. *Postepy w Kardiol Interwencyjnej/Advances in Interventional Cardiology* 2014;**10**(2):130–132. doi: 10.5114/pwki.2014.43522.
20. Mallery S. Endoscopic instrumentation. In: Shami VM, Kahaleh M (eds), *Endoscopic ultrasound*. New York: Springer, 2010:3–32.

Further reading

Dash D, Daggubati R. An update on clinical applications of intravascular ultrasound. *Journal of Cardiovascular Diseases & Diagnosis* 2015;**3**(5):215. doi: 10.4172/2329-9517.1000215.

North American Symptomatic Carotid Endarterectomy Trial Collaborators, Barnett HJM, Taylor DW, Haynes RB, Sackett DL, Peerless SJ, et al. Beneficial effect of carotid endarterectomy in symptomatic patients with high-grade carotid stenosis. *New England Journal of Medicine* 1991;**325**(7):445–453. doi: 10.1056/NEJM199108153250701.

CHAPTER 11
THE RESPIRATORY SYSTEM – LUNGS

The lungs   258
References   265

THE LUNGS

Previously, lung ultrasound was deemed unhelpful because ultrasound cannot penetrate air-containing structures. More recently, however, the number of applications for ultrasound of the pleura and lung fields has increased. Sonography is now used in evaluating pathology when fluid or a mass occupies the pleura, as well as changes to the lung caused by respiratory viruses, including coronaviruses. Ultrasound has several advantages over conventional radiography, such as the absence of radiation, the facility of real-time dynamic imaging and portability and, therefore, availability at the point of care or in the emergency setting.

Indications

- To distinguish between a pleural mass and fluid, since a loculated fluid pocket can be mistaken for a mass on a chest radiograph. Following radiographic appearances such as those shown in **Figure 11.1**, ultrasound can differentiate between consolidation and pleural effusion.[1]
- To assess diaphragmatic excursion, with the advantage of not employing ionising radiation.
- Thoracic assessment in the emergency situation for acute diagnosis of pneumothorax and haemothorax. Sonography has been shown to be of equivalent accuracy to chest radiography in detecting pneumothorax in patients with traumatic chest injury.[2]
- To identify the best entry point on the skin surface for the placement of a pleural drain.
- As a guide for thoracocentesis or tissue biopsy to obtain a sample for laboratory analysis where the causative factors are unknown. The British Thoracic Society (BTS) guidelines recommend that all thoracenteses be performed with ultrasound guidance.[3]
- Assessing progression of disease or response to treatment in patients with COVID-19 and other respiratory diseases.

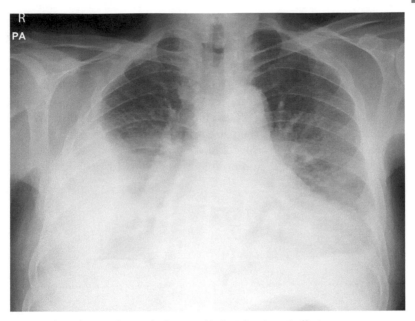

Figure 11.1 Chest radiograph showing likely right pleural effusion.

Patient preparation

No advance patient preparation is required. Attention to privacy and dignity must be paid while undressing. Infection control should be addressed if the patient has an infection or an open wound, or for invasive procedures such as drain insertion.

If available, a recent chest radiograph should be examined before the procedure to aid localisation of the pathology.

If possible, the patient should initially be in an upright sitting position, preferably on a backless stool to afford access from all sides. In this position, any free fluid will collect above the diaphragm where it is easier to see.

Imaging procedure

A small footprint probe is preferable to facilitate access between the ribs while permitting simultaneous imaging of the lung field and the diaphragm. Although resolution is not of paramount importance in chest sonography, as always, the selected frequency should be the highest possible for the depth under investigation, the optimum being 2.5–7.5 MHz.[4]

Having the patient sitting upright is the best position for imaging the posterior chest (**Figure 11.2**), whereas the anterior and lateral chest may be assessed in the lateral decubitus position (**Figure 11.3**). Raising the patient's arm above the head increases the rib space distance and facilitates scanning with the patient in erect or recumbent positions.[5] As well as ensuring all aspects of the lungs are easily accessible, the patient must be made comfortable enough not to move during any intervention.

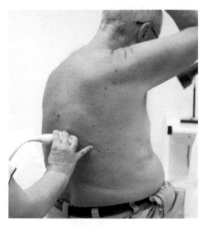

Figure 11.2 Patient in the erect position, to scan for a suspected pleural effusion.

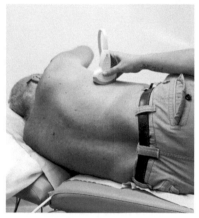

Figure 11.3 Patient in the left lateral decubitus position, for a lateral approach to the right lung.

A posterior approach is recommended, starting with the probe near the midline in an intercostal space just superior to the diaphragm. Pleural effusions usually pool above the diaphragm in the pleural recess, which descends much further posteriorly than anteriorly, so pleural effusions are often better imaged using a posterior approach. The probe is placed against the posterior aspect of the thorax near the midline at the intercostal space corresponding with the lower lobe and diaphragm, and moved along the intercostal space so that the pleura can be examined from the posterior and lateral aspects (**Figure 11.2**). The probe is moved higher to the next intercostal space, with the process repeated to trace the superior extent of an effusion or other pathology. During this procedure, the patient is asked to breathe deeply and hold their breath.

The patient is moved into a lateral decubitus position to facilitate lateral and anterior access (**Figure 11.3**). The anterior approach may be made using the right lobe of the liver and the spleen as acoustic windows for the respective right and left basal areas and diaphragmatic domes. This may be useful to see diaphragmatic excursion. The probe is placed on the anterior abdominal wall just below the costal cartilages and rib cage on either side of the trunk. Multiple views are obtained using a combination of transverse, parasagittal and oblique sections, with the transducer angled cranially. The patient should take deep breaths, during which the extent of movement can be assessed visually on the ultrasound monitor. M mode is useful to demonstrate and record any movement of a collapsed lung.

Image analysis

The first thing to observe is whether the lung parenchyma appears to slide with respiration.

Normal movement is demonstrated in **Figure 11.4**, where the differential movement of the deeper tissues against the stationary superficial tissues is known as the seashore sign. Also visible is the 'bat sign', which is the pattern made by the bright reflections from the ribs and pleura.[6]

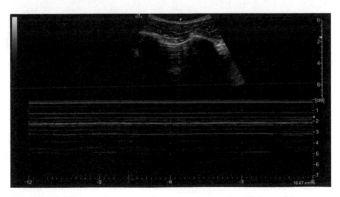

Figure 11.4 M mode trace of lung movement with breathing.

This is not particularly useful, other than for identification of anatomy, as it is present regardless of health or illness.

Lack of movement is suggestive of a pneumothorax, although it may represent other pathologies, so should be assessed in relation to the clinical history.[7] The 'lung point' may be visible in a partial pneumothorax; this is the point of transition between the area of lung sliding and its absence.[8]

Just deep to the ribs, the pleural line should be visible. Beyond this and parallel with it is the A-line, a reverberation artefact appearing as one or more bright horizontal lines (**Figure 11.5**). Visualisation of A-lines suggests that the lung is aerated, and the pleural surface is normal.[9] The lines appear smooth in the healthy lung.

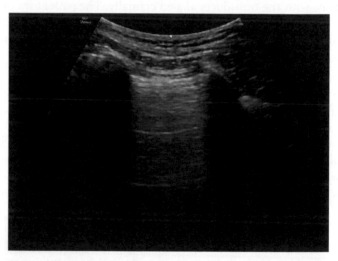

Figure 11.5 A-lines visible in a normal lung sonogram as reverberation artefacts below the pleural surface.

Vertical artefacts known as B-lines (formerly known as 'lung rockets', because they are comet tail artefacts) may be seen in **Figures 11.6** and **11.7**, extending from the pleural line perpendicularly into the lung parenchyma. More than three B-lines in two separate areas of lung are an abnormal finding and most likely due to interstitial oedema, which in turn has various underlying causes.[7] More B-lines usually suggest more severe disease.[10] They move as the lung slides during breathing.

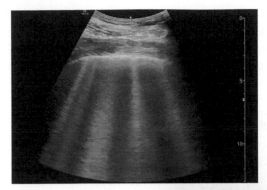

Figure 11.6 (left)
Chest sonogram of a patient, with known COVID-19 affecting the lungs. B-lines are visible.

Figure 11.7 (right)
Chest sonogram of the same patient, showing consolidation

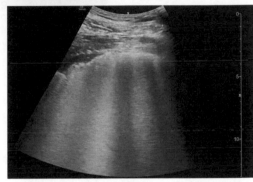

Consolidation may appear as subpleural hypoechoic tissue. It has a bright, irregular border with normally aerated lung, and this is known as the shred sign or fractal sign because of its irregularity. An example is seen in **Figure 11.7**.

Respiratory failure in COVID-19 or 'COVID lung' results in thickened pleura, small patchy areas of subpleural consolidation and interstitial oedema (**Figures 11.6** and **11.7**). The ultrasonic appearances are irregularity of the pleural line with multiple close B-lines and pulmonary consolidations (Jackson et al., 2021). Although these findings may be attributable to other lung diseases, there are subtle differentiating features that artificial intelligence (AI)-assisted scanning may be helpful in determining for a definitive diagnosis.[11] Ultrasound can be used to monitor patients over a period of time. Worsening of the condition produces an increasing number of B-lines, more consolidation affecting multiple areas of lung and potential air within the bronchi of consolidated lung, or 'air bronchograms'.[10] The reverse would apply in a recovering patient, and ultrasound can assess the response to treatment.

The usefulness of sonography in differentiation of pathological processes is illustrated by **Figure 11.8**, which shows consolidation of the left lung with a pleural effusion and ascites. This patient's chest radiograph would have very similar appearances to that in **Figure 11.1**.

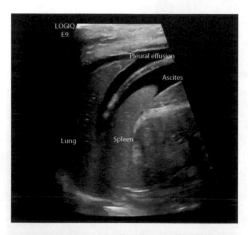

Figure 11.8 A sagittal section at the base of the left side of the chest, using a 9 MHz linear array transducer. This is a higher frequency than would generally be used, but, in this patient, it reveals excellent detail without compromising visualisation at depth.

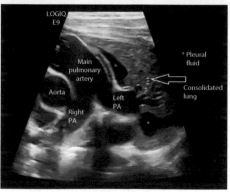

Figure 11.9 In the same patient as the previous image, this section shows chest anatomy, which is normally obscured by scattering from air in the lungs. PA, pulmonary artery.

In **Figure 11.9**, the chest anatomy is well demonstrated because of the lung consolidation and the extra pleural fluid, both of which transmit the sound well. The outflow tracts from the heart and the bifurcation of the pulmonary trunk are clearly seen.

REFERENCES

1. Prina E, Torres A, Carvalho CRR. Lung ultrasound in the evaluation of pleural effusion. *Jornal Brasileiro de Pneumologia* 2014;**40**(1):1–5. doi: 10.1590/S1806-37132014000100001.

2. Dulchavsky SA, Schwarz KL, Kirkpatrick AW, Billica RD, Williams DR, Diebel LN, et al. Prospective evaluation of thoracic ultrasound in the detection of pneumothorax. *Journal of Trauma* 2001;**50**(2):201–205. doi: 10.1097/00005373-200102000-00003.

3. Havelock T, Teoh R, Laws D, Gleeson F; BTS Pleural Disease Guideline Group. Pleural procedures and thoracic ultrasound: British Thoracic Society pleural disease guideline 2010. *Thorax* 2010;**65**(Suppl 2):ii61–ii76. doi: 10.1136/thx.2010.137026.

4. Soni NJ, Franco R, Velez MI, Schnobrich D, Dancel R, Restrepo MI, et al. Ultrasound in the diagnosis and management of pleural effusions. *Journal of Hospital Medicine* 2015;**10**(12):811–816. doi: 10.1002/jhm.2434.

5. Koh DM, Burke S, Davies N, Padley SP. Transthoracic US of the chest: Clinical uses and applications. *Radiographics* 2002;**22**(1):e1. doi: 10.1148/radiographics.22.1.g02jae1e1.

6. Bhoil R, Ahluwalia A, Chopra R, Surya M, Bhoil S. Signs and lines in lung ultrasound. *Journal of Ultrasonography* 2021;**21**(86):e255–e233. doi: 10.15557/JoU.2021.0036.

7. Taylor A, Anjum F, O'Rourke MC. *Thoracic and lung ultrasound.* [Updated 2021 Dec 8]. In: StatPearls [Internet]. Treasure Island (FL): StatPearls Publishing, 2021. Available at: https://www.ncbi.nlm.nih.gov/books/NBK500013.

8. Hew M, Tay TR. The efficacy of bedside chest ultrasound: From accuracy to outcomes. *European Respiratory Review* 2016;**25**(141):230–246. doi: 10.1183/16000617.0047-2016.

9. Jackson K, Butler R, Aujayeb A. Lung ultrasound in the COVID-19 pandemic. *Postgraduate Medical Journal* 2021;**97**(1143):34–39. doi: 10.1136/postgradmedj-2020-138137.

10. Smith MJ, Hayward SA, Innes SM, Miller ASC. Point-of-care lung ultrasound in patients with COVID-19 – a narrative review. *Anaesthesia* 2020;**75**(8):1096–1104. doi: 10.1111/anae.15082.

11. Arntfield R, VanBerlo B, Alaifan T, Phelps N, White M, Chaudhary R, et al. Development of a deep learning classifier to accurately distinguish COVID-19 from look-a-like pathology on lung ultrasound. *medRxiv* 2020. doi: 10.1101/2020.10.13.20212258.

CHAPTER 12

THE CENTRAL NERVOUS SYSTEM – EYE AND BRAIN

Ocular ultrasound   268

The neonatal brain   272

References   278

OCULAR ULTRASOUND

Ultrasound is a fast, painless, non-invasive method of examining the soft tissue within the orbits. As ultrasound does not travel well through bone, it is not possible to assess the bony orbit or beyond. However, ocular ultrasound comes into its own in cases of trauma to the eye, when swelling of the eyelids renders direct visualisation using an ophthalmoscope impossible.

Because the eye is a superficial structure, an electronic linear array transducer is the probe of choice. The highest available frequency should be used, at least 7.5–10 MHz, to give good resolution with adequate penetration to the 4 cm depth that is required for this examination. Some units may have a dedicated ophthalmic probe, which is small and light, facilitating delicate movements more easily.

Indications

Sonography is the examination of choice for the eye following trauma to investigate for possible retinal detachment, haemorrhage, localisation of foreign bodies or globe rupture. It can also enable measurement of the diameter of the optic nerve sheath in patients with suspected raised intracranial pressure and may aid emergency diagnosis and management.[1]

Ultrasound is also used for assessment of the eye in circumstances when the lens and/or the aqueous and vitreous substances are opaque and do not permit direct examination with an ophthalmoscope, for instance corneal oedema, vitreous haemorrhage or unilateral cataracts, which may be associated with intraocular tumour.

Patient preparation

The patient should lie supine, with the head resting on a low pillow, and be reassured that the procedure will not cause pain or damage to the eye. Both eyes should be scanned through closed eyelids. If conscious, the patient should be asked to keep the eyes still and to focus on a fixed point on the ceiling, or to look straight ahead, and to then close the eyes, keeping the pupils fixed in this position as far as possible until instructed otherwise.

Ultrasonic gel is not normally detrimental to the tissues of the eye, but of course stringent infection control measures should be used. There is evidence to suggest that ultrasound gel can cause harm if in contact with mucous membranes[2] and bacterial infection can lead to visual impairment following ophthalmic surgery,[3] so single-use sterile gel sachets should be used. Sufficient gel should be placed on the transducer face so that, when the probe is offered gently to the eye, it is not in contact with the eyelid itself; any pressure on the eye should be minimised, particularly after trauma. The exposure should be limited, especially if Doppler ultrasound is used, because of the sensitivity of eye tissue.

Imaging procedure

During this procedure, both eyes are examined for comparison. The initial probe placement should demonstrate a cross-section through the centre of the eye.

A series of transverse sections of the entire eye is acquired, demonstrating on each image both anterior and posterior borders of the eye and the area posterior to the eye. From the initial scanning position, the probe is gently moved and angled both cranially and caudally, with the patient encouraged to keep the eye closed and motionless during the procedure (**Figure 12.1**).

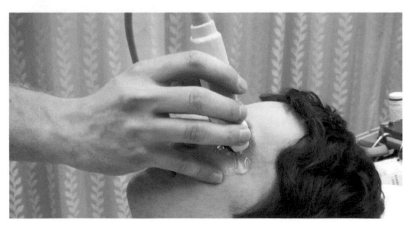

Figure 12.1 Probe position for ocular sonography.

Following this initial evaluation, the patient is asked to move the eye gently as if looking first to the left and then to the right, in turn. Movement in the interior of the eye is observed and recorded.

Colourflow Doppler may be employed in the investigation of vascular disease and tumour blood supply.

Image analysis

Both eyes should appear as roughly spherical structures. The transverse section through the normal eye as demonstrated in **Figures 12.2** and **12.3** shows the eyelid, cornea, anterior chamber and posterior chamber. The posterior chamber is behind the lens and is occupied by the vitreous body, or vitreous humour, sometimes known simply as the vitreous.

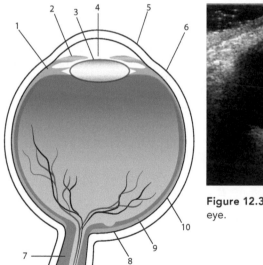

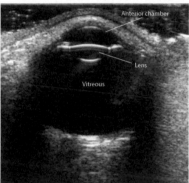

Figure 12.3 Sonogram of a normal eye.

Figure 12.2 Diagrammatic section through the normal eye: (1) ciliary body (muscle); (2) iris; (3) lens; (4) anterior chamber and pupil; (5) cornea; (6) sclera (continuous with cornea); (7) optic nerve, travelling slightly medially; (8) fovea; (9) retina; and (10) choroid.

The cornea is seen as a thin hypoechoic layer parallel to the eyelid. The anterior chamber is filled with anechoic fluid and is bordered by the cornea, iris and the anterior reflection of the lens capsule. The normal lens is anechoic and the normal vitreous body is relatively anechoic in a young healthy eye. The evaluation of the retrobulbar area includes the optic nerve, extraocular muscles and bony orbit. Each optic nerve may be demonstrated as a hypoechoic structure approximately 2–3 mm thick, directed medially from the posterior aspect of the globe.

Sonographically, the normal retina cannot be differentiated from the other choroidal layers,[4] as shown in **Figure 12.3**. However, a detached retina can be diagnosed in the presence of an undulating hyperechoic membrane within the globe (**Figures 12.4** and **12.5**).

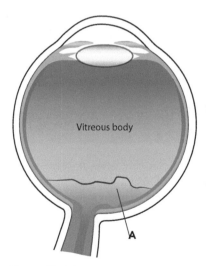

Figure 12.4 Diagrammatic section of the eye, showing an area of retinal detachment (A).

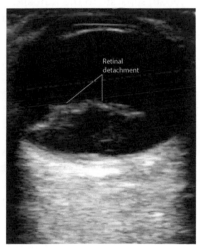

Figure 12.5 Sonogram of an eye, showing a detached retina.

Intraocular foreign bodies can be identified as bright hyperechoic areas. Ultrasound artefacts such as acoustic shadowing or reverberation artefacts in the usually clear vitreous humour may help differentiate foreign materials (**Figure 12.6**).

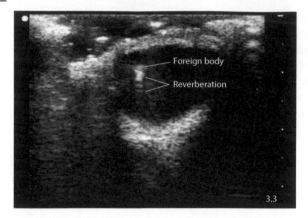

Foreign body

Reverberation

Figure 12.6
Sonogram of the eye, showing a foreign body; the blue-coloured overlay has been added for clarity.

Vitreous haemorrhage may be seen as a hyperechoic area within the eyeball, separate to the wall and moving with eye movements. As with haemorrhage elsewhere in the body, sonographic appearances may vary with the duration and progress of clot formation.

Ophthalmic tumours appear as hyperechoic masses, generally attached to the wall and moving with eye movements.

THE NEONATAL BRAIN

Newborn babies and small infants have relatively large, poorly ossified heads compared with the rest of the body. This unique anatomical constellation makes them particularly vulnerable to brain injuries, but also facilitates assessment of the brain using sonography. Additionally, in preterm infants at the edge of viability the brain is very immature, magnifying the risks of serious brain injury, leading to death or long-term neurodevelopmental problems. Sonographic assessment of the brain becomes crucial in the management of these babies.

Indications

Neonatal cranial sonography is used to screen for acquired brain injuries such as acute haemorrhage, especially in the ventricles. More recently the scope has been extended to include acute non-haemorrhagic lesions of the brain such as periventricular leukomalacia, hypoxic-ischaemic encephalopathy or ischaemic stroke.[5] In addition, congenital anomalies are increasingly being detected using ultrasound, aiding the diagnostic approach in newborns with complex problems, for example septo-optic dysplasia. With the advent of improved transducer technology and better techniques, screening for more deeply sited lesions in other areas of the brain, for example the cerebellum, has also become possible. Sonography is increasingly used instead of computed tomography (CT) or magnetic resonance imaging (MRI) for monitoring established conditions with or without continuing treatment, for example hydrocephalus with shunt.

Patient preparation

The utmost hand hygiene should always be observed when examining newborns.[6] Before and after examining the newborn, the probe and cable should be cleaned with a manufacturer-approved wipe soaked in an alcohol-free detergent.[5]

Newborn babies are very susceptible to cold and every effort should be made to minimise heat loss during the examination. Single-use sterile gel sachets should be used.[2] If necessary, the gel can be warmed.

No specific preparation of the patient is required. Newborns can easily be examined in an open cot or incubator, although access to the head might be limited depending on gestation at birth, their general condition, other diagnostic or therapeutic interventions and bed space. Good communication with the neonatal team looking after the newborn will help avoid safety hazards and allow for more efficient imaging.

Imaging procedure

A phased (sector) array transducer with a small footprint and a frequency of 10–12 MHz is used. This has the advantage of electronic beam steering without moving the probe.

The sonographer should be confident in scanning a baby who is lying prone or supine and from either side of the cot or incubator as conditions dictate. The probe is placed gently on the anterior fontanelle (**Figures 12.7** and **12.8**). Starting in the coronal axis, six standard coronal images, including the one in **Figure 12.9**, are obtained by angling the probe sequentially anteriorly and posteriorly along the lines superimposed on **Figures 12.8** and **12.10**.

The probe is then rotated 90° into the sagittal plane to acquire a midline sagittal view such as that in **Figure 12.10**. Parasagittal images of each hemisphere are then obtained by angling the probe to the left and right, towards the Sylvian fissures, along the planes illustrated by the lines in **Figures 12.7** and **12.9**.

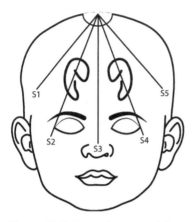

Figure 12.7 Front elevation of the head, with the lines S1 to S5 showing the range of probe angulations for sagittal and parasagittal planes.

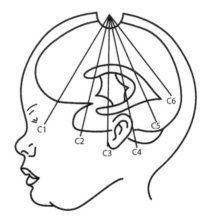

Figure 12.8 Diagram of a midline sagittal section. The lines C1 to C6 indicate the range of probe angulations for coronal plane imaging.

Additional views may be required according to the initial request or clinical question, the age of the baby, pathological findings and judgement of the sonographer. These may be possible through the same or other fontanelles as appropriate.[5,7]

For transaxial imaging, the probe is placed against the temporoparietal bone to acquire two sections in the transaxial plane, one at the level of the cerebral peduncles, the second showing the lateral ventricles.

Normal anatomy and any pathology must be recorded in two planes and the whole examination documented.

Image analysis

The ultrasound images in **Figures 12.9** and **12.10** show two key sections, with the lines on each representing the planes of scanning to achieve the additional sections of the other. Hence this coronal section shows the possible sagittal planes of scan, whereas the sagittal shows the coronal planes. An examination should comprise between three and seven lines of imaging in both the coronal and the sagittal planes along with dynamic scanning.

The coronal series should contain images of the frontal lobes, frontal ventricular horns, the bodies of the lateral ventricles with the foramen of Monro and the third ventricle, the occipital horns of the lateral ventricles and the occipital lobes.

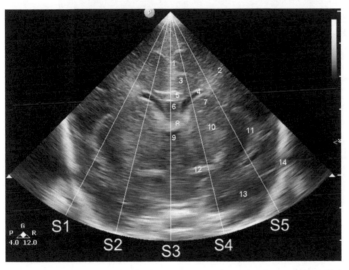

Figure 12.9 A coronal section at the level of the third ventricle and thalami.

1. Interhemispheric fissure
2. Parietal lobe
3. Cingulate gyrus
4. Left lateral ventricle
5. Corpus callosum
6. Cavum septum pellucidum
7. Caudate nucleus
8. Choroid plexus, extending through the foramina of Monro

9. Third ventricle
10. Thalamus
11. Sylvian fissure
12. Medial cerebral artery
13. Temporal lobe
14. Temporal fontanelle.

A coronal section of the brain is shown on **Figure 12.9**, taken through the plane C3 of **Figure 12.10**. The five standard sagittal planes, S1 to S5, are demonstrated.

The midline sagittal section of the brain in **Figure 12.10** is taken through the plane S3 of **Figure 12.9**. The lines show the six standard coronal planes, C1–C6.

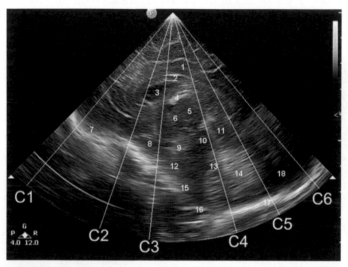

Figure 12.10 A sagittal section of the brain. The anterior part of the brain is to the left of the image.

1. Cingulate gyrus
2. Corpus callosum
3. Cavum septum pellucidum
4. Fornix
5. Thalamus
6. Third ventricle
7. Frontal base of the skull
8. Interpeduncular fossa
9. Mesencephalon
10. Aqueduct
11. Quadrigeminal cistern
12. Pons
13. Fourth ventricle
14. Cerebellum
15. Medulla oblongata
16. Foramen magnum
17. Occipital base of the skull
18. Cisterna magna.

A coronal section through the brain of a premature infant, born at 30 weeks' gestation, is demonstrated in **Figure 12.11**. This shows the posterior horns of the lateral ventricles, which are dilated. There is associated intraventricular haemorrhage (IVH), in this case grade 3.[8] Premature babies have a high risk of IVH and are routinely monitored for this condition.

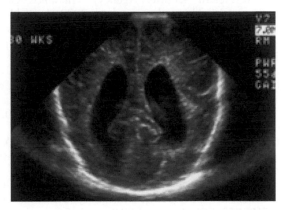

Figure 12.11 A coronal section, taken through the plane C4 of **Figure 12.10**.

IVH is graded using the following criteria:
- Grade 1: haemorrhage confined to the subependymal matrix. Seen as anechoic area filling the caudate nucleus (**Figure 12.9**).
- Grade 2: haemorrhage filling less than half of the ventricular system.
- Grade 3: haemorrhage filling over half of the ventricle, with associated ventriculomegaly.
- Grade 4: haemorrhage extending beyond the ventricles into the brain parenchyma.

REFERENCES

1. Kilker BA, Holst JM, Hoffmann B. Bedside ocular ultrasound in the emergency department. *European Journal of Emergency Medicine* 2014;**21**(4):246–253. doi: 10.1097/MEJ.0000000000000070.
2. UKHSA (UK Health Security Agency). *Guidance. Good infection prevention practice: Using ultrasound gel*, 2022. Available at: https://www.gov.uk/government/publications/ultrasound-gel-good-infection-prevention-practice/good-infection-prevention-practice-using-ultrasound-gel.
3. Lind C, Olsen K, Angelsen NK, Krefting EA, Fossen K, Gravningen K, Clinical course, treatment and visual outcome of an outbreak of *Burkholderia contaminans* endophthalmitis following cataract surgery. *Journal of Ophthalmic Inflammation and Infection* 2021;**11**(1):12. doi: 10.1186/s12348-021-00242-6.
4. Situ-LaCasse E, Adhikari SR. *Ocular emergencies*. Irving, TX: American College of Emergency Physicians, 2020. Available at: https://www.acep.org/sonoguide/smparts_ocular.html.
5. AIUM practice parameter for the performance of neurosonography in neonates and infants. *Journal of Ultrasound in Medicine* 2020;**39**(5):E57–E61. doi: 10.1002/jum.15264.
6. Sax H, Allegranzi B, Uçkay I, Larson E, Boyce J, Pittet D. 'My five moments for hand hygiene': A user-centred design approach to understand, train, monitor and report hand hygiene. *Journal of Hospital Infection* 2007;**67**(1):9–21. doi: 10.1016/j.jhin.2007.06.004.
7. Lowe LH, Bailey Z. State-of-the-art cranial sonography: Part 1, modern techniques and image interpretation. *American Journal of Roentgenology* 2011;**196**(5):1028–1033. doi: 10.2214/AJR.10.6160.
8. Brouwer MJ, de Vries LS, Groenendaal F, Koopman C, Pistorius LR, Mulder EJH, et al. New reference values for the neonatal cerebral ventricles. *Radiology* 2012;**262**(1):224–233. doi: 10.1148/radiol.11110334.

Further reading

Rennie JM, Hagmann CF, Robertson NJ, (eds.). *Neonatal cerebral investigation*. 2nd edn. Cambridge: Cambridge University Press, 2008.

CHAPTER 13

MUSCULOSKELETAL ULTRASOUND

The shoulder   280
The elbow   285
The wrist and hand   289
The paediatric hip joint   294
The knee   303
The ankle and foot   308
Ultrasound-guided interventions   314
References   318

THE SHOULDER

Ultrasound has been established as an effective imaging method in the musculoskeletal system. Besides the non-ionising nature of ultrasound, the main advantages include the ability to perform dynamic examinations, to conduct side-by-side comparisons on the spot and to guide interventions such as fluid aspirations or cavity injections.

The shoulder joint is a synovial ball-and-socket joint made up of the scapula's glenoid cavity and the articular surface of the humeral head. It has a wide range of movements and relies on the support of the rotator cuff muscles for stability.

Indications

Ultrasound is especially useful in the shoulder due to the high incidence of rotator cuff disorders and ease of access. The four rotator cuff muscles are: the subscapularis muscle at the anterior aspect of the shoulder; the supraspinatus muscle at its superior aspect; and the infraspinatus muscle and teres minor muscle, which are both situated at the posterior aspect.

Patients showing progressive onset of shoulder pain and night pain are typically referred for an ultrasound examination. These symptoms are most common in patients aged over 50 years and slightly predominate in women.[1]

If the patient presents with persistent pain in the anterolateral aspect of the shoulder, ultrasound can be useful for the diagnosis of: impingement syndrome; rotator cuff tendinopathy or tear; joint effusion and bursal fluid; acromioclavicular (AC) joint pathology; and biceps muscle injury. In posterior shoulder pain, ultrasound can be useful to diagnose rotator cuff tendinopathy or tears and posterior labrum lesions. Many of these symptoms are linked with sports injuries or arise as a result of work-related strain.[2]

Patient preparation

As always, the procedure should be fully explained to the patient before starting.

Clothing around the shoulder area should be removed. Care is required during the ultrasound examination, as the patient is asked to move and rotate the arm, which can increase pain in the shoulder and, consequently, reduce shoulder movements.

After the examination, ask if the patient needs help dressing; assistance with clothing may be required due to the shoulder symptoms.

Imaging procedure

The patient should be seated on a revolving stool at a height that is comfortable for the sonographer, who should be behind the patient, allowing more probe stability and less hand fatigue. The examination is performed using a high-frequency (>7.5 MHz) linear array transducer.

A systematic, step-by-step examination is performed with the first step starting with the long head of the biceps tendon. This is examined in the longitudinal and transverse planes, with the patient's forearm and hand resting in a supinated position on the thigh.

The patient is then asked to externally rotate the arm, to study the subscapularis tendon in longitudinal and transverse planes from the lesser tuberosity to the coracoid process.

The third step requires a manoeuvre to expose the supraspinatus tendon anteriorly beneath the acromion. The goal is to produce internal rotation and hyperextension, by asking the patient to place the arm behind their back (**Figure 13.1**). The supraspinatus tendon should be

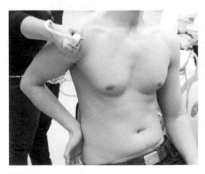

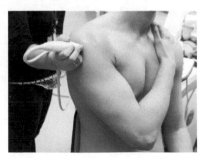

Figure 13.1 Taking the patient's hand behind the back facilitates examination of the supraspinatus tendon.

Figure 13.2 Placing the hand on the opposite shoulder facilitates viewing the infraspinatus and teres minor muscles and tendons of the posterior part of the rotator cuff.

evaluated from the superior facet of the greater tuberosity to the acromion, along both its long and short axes.

In the final step, the patient places the hand on the opposite shoulder to internally rotate the humerus (**Figure 13.2**) and the transducer is placed over the posterior aspect of the glenohumeral joint, to view the infraspinatus and teres minor muscles and tendons. The acromioclavicular joint can then be viewed by placing the transducer in the coronal plane, sweeping anteriorly and posteriorly over the joint during the examination.

Dynamic assessment should always be performed for rotator cuff impingement, so that the greater tuberosity and acromion process are visualised in the same field of view.

Image analysis

The first structure to be identified is the biceps tendon, located in the bicipital groove and used as a reference landmark (**Figure 13.3**). As with all ultrasound examinations, it is vital for the operator to understand both the anatomy of the part under examination and the artefactual errors that may be caused by poor technique. The latter is illustrated by the two transverse images of the biceps tendon in the shoulder (**Figures 13.4 and 13.5**).

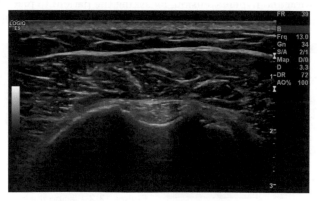

Figure 13.3 The long head of biceps in transverse section. The tendon appears as an oval hyperechoic (bright) structure located in the bicipital groove, between the greater and lesser tuberosities.

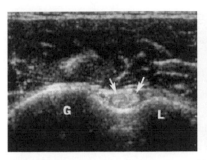
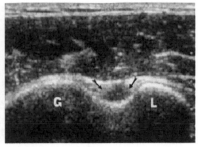

Figures 13.4 and 13.5 Comparison of biceps tendon appearances. The letters 'G' and 'L' indicate the greater and lesser trochanters, with the biceps tendon between them.

In **Figure 13.4**, the tendon (white arrows) appears normal, but in **Figure 13.5** the same tendon appears hypoechoic (black arrows). The apparent difference in echodensity is known as anisotropy and is an artefactual appearance caused by poor technique. This is due to a slight angulation of the probe in **Figure 13.5**, evidenced by close inspection of the superficial tissues, and resulting in a non-planar reflection and failure to capture all the echoes from the tendon. This slight angulation error could lead to a false diagnosis of tendon pathology in the unwary.

The subscapularis tendon (**Figure 13.6**) appears as a hyperechoic band that follows the contour of the lesser tuberosity. Anterior to the tendon the deltoid muscle can be observed. The supraspinatus tendon is recognisable by the parallel and fine fibril pattern, with a convex superior margin (**Figure 13.7**). The thin anechoic line corresponds to the normal subacromial–subdeltoid bursa.

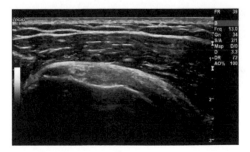

Figure 13.6 Longitudinal view of the subscapularis tendon, medial to the proximal portion of the biceps tendon.

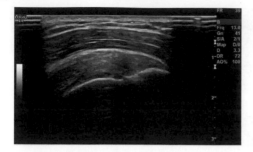

Figure 13.7 Longitudinal view of the supraspinatus tendon.

The infraspinatus tendon appears hyperechoic centrally with hypoechoic tendon fibres superiorly and inferiorly (**Figure 13.8**). It inserts into the middle facet of the greater tuberosity.

The articular surfaces of the AC joint are smooth and rounded, with the joint space identified as the hypoechoic gap between them (**Figure 13.9**). Adjacent bony structures show posterior acoustic shadowing.

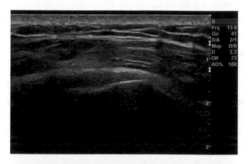

Figure 13.8 Longitudinal view of the infraspinatus tendon.

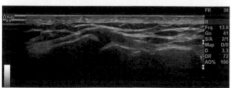

Figure 13.9 AC joint.

THE ELBOW

Ultrasound has become increasingly important in the evaluation of the complex anatomy of the elbow, being readily available and more cost-effective than magnetic resonance imaging (MRI). It has high sensitivity and specificity for medial and lateral epicondylitis, also known as golfer's and tennis elbow respectively. Ultrasound can detect biceps and triceps tendon tears, whether partial or complete, bursitis and lesions of the ulnar, radial or median nerve.

Indications

Elbow ultrasound is used in the investigation of:

- lateral pain, which is increased with active extension of the wrist;
- posterior pain, particularly in the presence of olecranon bursitis, or student's elbow and triceps tendinosis or tear;
- medial pain, in the suspicion of medial epicondylitis, worsened by resisted forearm pronation and wrist flexion, or in the assessment of entrapment or subluxation of the ulnar nerve;
- anterior pain, related to biceps tendinosis or tear.

Patient preparation

The patient should be seated facing the sonographer and the elbow placed on an examination table, or the patient may lie supine on the examination table.

Imaging procedure

A high-frequency (at least 10 MHz) linear array transducer is used, and colourflow or power Doppler should be available to assess vascularity in tendinopathy.

To evaluate the anterior aspect of the elbow, the joint is supported by a pillow and extended, with the hand in supine position. The probe is placed in the long axis over the anterior elbow (**Figure 13.10**). This allows the study of the brachialis muscle, median nerve, coronoid fossa, anterior elbow process and trochlea on the medial (ulnar) side. More laterally, it is possible to evaluate the biceps tendon, the capitellum and radial head (**Figure 13.12**). Transverse imaging should also be performed.

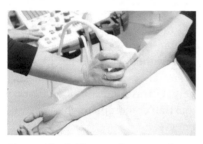

Figure 13.10 The initial position for elbow ultrasound, with the arm and hand supinated.

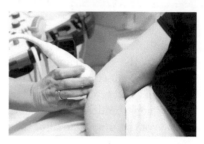

Figure 13.11 Position for scanning the posterior aspect of the elbow.

In the evaluation of the lateral aspect of the elbow, the joint should be flexed at 90°. The superior edge of the probe is then oriented to the lateral epicondyle and the probe is placed longitudinally to visualise the common extensor tendon. In the proximal portion of the tendon, transverse plane imaging may improve the accuracy of the examination.

For the medial aspect, the elbow is extended and the patient leans towards the side with the forearm in external rotation. The probe is oriented to the medial epicondyle, in a coronal plane, and the common flexor tendon appears in its long axis.

The posterior aspect of the elbow is studied with the elbow flexed at 90° with the palm resting on the table (**Figure 13.11**). Proximal to the olecranon, the triceps muscle and tendon should be evaluated in long and short axis (**Figure 13.12**). Located deep to triceps, the olecranon fossa and posterior recess should also be examined.

To study the cubital tunnel, the probe is placed parallel to the olecranon and the medial epicondyle, and the ulnar nerve is examined from the distal arm through the forearm in transverse sections. Dynamic evaluation should be performed to detect the presence of intra-articular fluid or nerve instability.[3]

Image analysis

The biceps muscle is seen in the anterior aspect of the elbow and superior to the joint. It lies deep to the subcutaneous tissue surrounded by the brachial fascia, appearing as a bipennate muscle with a central hyperechoic layer. **Figure 13.13** shows the distal biceps tendon more inferiorly, where it may appear hypoechoic due to anisotropy, an artefactual appearance explained in **Figures 13.4** and **13.5**. This artefact is a common appearance in the distal biceps tendon, since it has an oblique course from surface to depth to insert in the bicipital tuberosity. Just deep to this, the typical hypoechoic appearance of the brachialis muscle is seen, with intervening hyperechoic fibroadipose septa. Deep in the muscle, the coronoid fossa is visible as a prominent concavity in the distal humerus, with a triangular hyperechoic intracapsular fat pad. The anterior aspect of the bones forming the joint can be seen, with a thin layer (~2 mm) of hypoechoic articular cartilage at their surfaces.

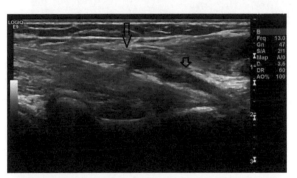

Figure 13.12
The distal biceps tendon (arrowed).

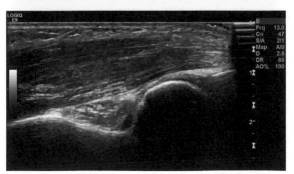

Figure 13.13
The triceps tendon demonstrated at the posterior aspect of the elbow.

The distal triceps tendon appears hyperechoic and typically exhibits striations in its insertion in the olecranon (**Figure 13.13**).

Deeper, at the posterior aspect of the humeral shaft, a pronounced concavity is observed, the olecranon fossa, filled with the hyperechoic posterior fat pad. More distally, the olecranon process should be examined, using slight pressure with the transducer to assess for the presence of bursitis.

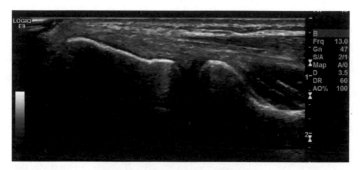

Figure 13.14 The common extensor tendon origin.

The common extensor tendon origin appears as a beak-shaped hyperechoic structure located between the subcutaneous tissue and the lateral ulnar collateral ligament (**Figure 13.14**). The common flexor tendon inserts in the medial epicondyle and appears shorter than the common extensor tendon (**Figure 13.15**). Both tendons have a normal fibrillar pattern. Due to this pattern, it is sometimes difficult to differentiate the lateral ulnar collateral ligament and the extensor tendon.

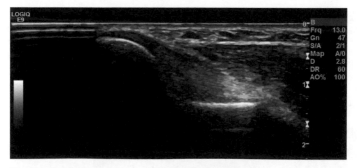

Figure 13.15 The common flexor tendon origin.

THE WRIST AND HAND

High-resolution and real-time greyscale imaging make ultrasound the optimum imaging modality to evaluate small and superficial ligaments of the wrist. It has the advantages of dynamic study of tendon movement in the tendon sheaths and the possibility of vascular assessment using colourflow Doppler ultrasound. In combination with standard radiographs, ultrasound is a reliable tool for the diagnosis of wrist abnormalities and it is gradually achieving the same results as MRI,[4] with particular usefulness for real-time guidance during therapeutic procedures.

Indications

- When tenosynovitis and other tendinopathies are suspected, for example, De Quervain's tenosynovitis, a condition that affects the tendons of the first compartment and its retinaculum, and other abnormalities in tendons, such as tears.
- Carpal and ulnar tunnel syndromes: by evaluating nerve swelling and the demonstration of blood flow using power Doppler.
- Detection of inflammatory joint disease or infection, such as rheumatoid arthritis and psoriatic arthritis.
- Soft-tissue masses of the wrist and hand.[5]

Patient preparation

The patient's history should be carefully investigated to consider systemic joint disease, sporting or occupational activities, as well as local trauma. Wrist ultrasound is typically performed with the patient seated and the hand resting on the examination table.

Imaging procedure

Using a high-frequency linear array transducer of at least 10 MHz, sonographic evaluation starts with the palm facing the examination table (**Figure 13.16**). On the dorsal side, the wrist is divided into six synovial compartments. The bony landmark used is Lister's tubercule in the transverse plane, separating the second and third compartments.

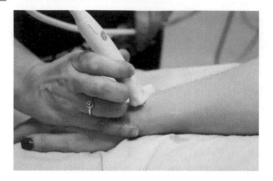

Figure 13.16 Technique for a transverse section of the posterior aspect of the wrist, to image the extensor tendons.

Lateral to Lister's tubercule, the second compartment is identified, consisting of the extensor carpi radialis longus and brevis tendons. Placing the wrist in a halfway position between pronation and supination and moving the transducer to the lateral aspect of the radial edge of the dorsal wrist, the first compartment is examined. This contains the abductor pollicis longus and extensor pollicis brevis tendons. The retinaculum should be identified and examined for any sign of thickening.

The probe is placed at Lister's tubercle again and moved medially to identify the third compartment, containing the extensor pollicis longus tendon. Distally, this tendon crosses anterior to the tendons of the second compartment. The probe is moved medially to examine the fourth and fifth compartment in the mid-dorsal wrist. Within the fourth compartment are the four extensor digitorum tendons and the extensor indicis tendon, whilst the fifth contains the extensor digiti minimi tendon.

To individualise each tendon, sequential flexion and extension of the fingers should be performed, with the wrist in slight radial deviation. Typically, the extensor digiti minimi is identified anteriorly to the articular cartilage of the ulnar head. The sixth compartment consists of the extensor carpi ulnaris tendon lying on the medial aspect of the ulnar head.

For each compartment, the probe is swept cranially in the transverse plane up to the muscle-tendon junction and then down to the distal insertion.

Finally, the wrist is placed on the examination table with the hand supinated. The probe is placed on the palmar aspect of the wrist in the transverse plane, just proximal to the carpal tunnel (**Figure 13.17**), whose key anatomical structure is the flexor retinaculum. This contains the flexor pollicis longus (FPL) tendon, the four flexor digitorum profundus tendons, the four flexor digitorum superficialis tendons and the median nerve. Imaging in longitudinal planes may help in dynamic evaluation and to assess the extent of any anatomical change (**Figure 13.18**).

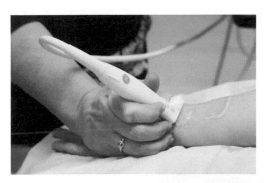

Figure 13.17 Technique for a transverse section of the anterior aspect of the wrist, to image the carpal tunnel.

Figure 13.18 Technique for a longitudinal section of the anterior aspect of the wrist.

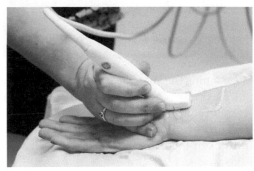

Image analysis

Normal tendons of the wrist display the following characteristics:

- They are hyperechoic, appearing relatively bright.
- They are longitudinally oriented, with a fibrillar pattern, reflecting the presence of highly reflective (hyperechoic) collagen fibre bundles surrounded by a hypoechoic matrix.
- In transverse plane, tendons appear as oval structures with a pinpoint pattern of echoes.
- Tendon sheaths are observed as hypoechoic lines.
- The extensor tendon sheaths typically contain a small amount of anechoic fluid.

The flexor retinaculum appears as a thin slightly convex band of 1 to 1.5 mm thickness. Both flexor and extensor retinacula can be observed as hypoechoic bands and their bony insertions can be appreciated. **Figure 13.19** shows the second and third extensor compartments separated by Lister's tubercle (the triangular dorsal tubercle of the radius). This image corresponds to the positioning in **Figure 13.16**.

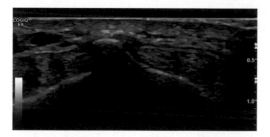

Figure 13.19
Dorsal aspect of the wrist.

Scanning the anterior aspect of the wrist in transverse section **(Figure 13.20,** position as in **Figure 13.17)** shows the scapholunate joint in the carpal tunnel. A longitudinal scan of the anterior aspect of the wrist **(Figure 13.21,** position as in **Figure 13.18)** shows the tendons of the flexor carpi radialis and the flexor pollicis longus.

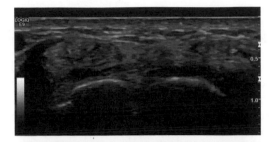

Figure 13.20
Anterior aspect of
the wrist.

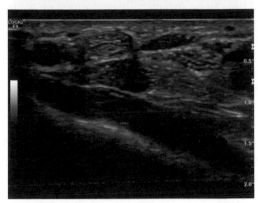

Figure 13.21
Longitudinal scan of
the wrist.

It may be necessary to tilt the probe to examine the tendons properly and avoid anisotropy. Dynamic and long axis imaging may help to individualise each tendon and to assess integrity. Each structure should be examined for possible thickening proximally and distally to the carpal tunnel.

The median nerve runs superficial to and parallel with the flexor tendons, and medial to the FPL tendon. Deep to the flexor retinaculum, it is identified by its hypoechoic nerve fascicles, showing a round or oval shape.

If there is suspicion of inflammatory arthritis, the dorsal radiocarpal, midcarpal, metacarpophalangeal and, if symptomatic, proximal interphalangeal joints can be evaluated for effusion, synovial hypertrophy and bony erosions. Other joints of the wrist and hand are similarly evaluated as clinically indicated.[6–8]

THE PAEDIATRIC HIP JOINT

Ultrasound is a first-line investigation of the neonatal hip, and should be used in imaging of paediatric hips whenever possible to reduce the radiation dose to this particularly radiosensitive section of the population. It is unlikely that ultrasound will completely replace radiographs in paediatric hip examination, although its use is expanding. Sonographic assessment of the neonatal hip can be successfully performed up to the age of 6 months, sometimes even up to 10–12 months, depending on the degree of ossification of the capital femoral epiphysis. Ultrasound allows visualisation of cartilaginous as well as ossified areas of the bone that cannot be seen on radiographic imaging, it shows the joint capsule and tissue layers and allows a dynamic examination to be undertaken.

Indications

The main indication for hip ultrasound is in the diagnosis and monitoring of developmental dysplasia of the hip (DDH). This was previously known as congenital dislocation of the hip; however, it is now acknowledged as a progressive condition, variable in manifestation and not always detectable at birth.[9] Its causes can be classified as follows:

- **Physiological**: a combination of genetic factors and maternal hormones. The majority of children with DDH have ligamentous laxity, which predisposes to hip instability.
- **Mechanical**: a result of positional influences in utero, for example breech presentation, oligohydramnios and multiple pregnancies.

Babies are examined for this condition at birth and at 6–8 weeks using the Barlow and Ortalani tests, which are physical manoeuvres to assess laxity in the joint.[10,11]

Other uses of paediatric hip ultrasound are to demonstrate hip joint effusion, which may be due to transient synovitis or juvenile idiopathic arthritis, and occasionally to visualise Legge–Calve–Perthes disease (often abbreviated to LCPD or simply to Perthes' disease) or a slipped capital femoral epiphysis, although it is not the first line of investigation for either of these.

Patient preparation

If possible, the infant should attend for the examination having been fed and changed. The area between the waist and the knees should be uncovered. The nappy may be left in place and unfastened one side at a time. A full explanation of the examination and the need to keep the baby relaxed and still should be given to the parent or carer to gain their cooperation.

Imaging procedure

Although various methods of infant hip sonography have been described, the Graf technique[12] is the most widely used sonographic method of examining neonatal hips for DDH in Europe. For this, the baby is placed on their side, using a positioning device if available. Otherwise the carer is asked to hold the baby's shoulder and knees, keeping the baby's back as vertical as possible to ensure that the baby does not roll from position. The knees should be bent and the hip being examined held in slight internal rotation. Ultrasound gel is applied and a linear array transducer with a frequency of at least 7.5 MHz is placed over the greater trochanter in the coronal plane It is crucial that the probe be held vertical,[13] as shown in **Figure 13.22**; some centres use a clamp to maintain the probe in true vertical.

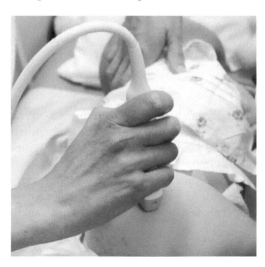

Figure 13.22 A baby being scanned to obtain a coronal section of the hip.

Figure 13.23 A standard coronal view, to assess the depth and maturity of the acetabulum, and whether the femoral head is centred within the acetabulum.

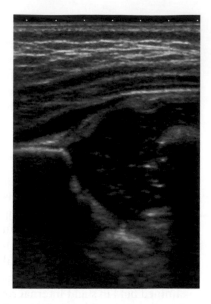

A modification to the Graf technique includes a dynamic assessment of the hip to assess the stability of the femoral head within the acetabulum under stress. Stress views are obtained by directing pressure posteriorly with the femur in 90° of flexion and maximum adduction, as in the Barlow manoeuvre, although it is important to note that the hip joints should be classified without stress.[13] Images of any stress views should be recorded. In difficult cases, the transverse view may also be used to assess the location of the femoral head.

Image analysis

The Graf technique as demonstrated in **Figure 13.22** produces a coronal section (**Figure 13.23**) on which a series of landmarks can be identified, as labelled in **Figure 13.24**. These landmarks are connected by lines, whose angles can be measured (**Figure 13.25**).

These landmarks should be identifiable on an image of diagnostic quality. One exception to this rule is a decentred hip; if the femoral head is dislocated, the standard plane cannot be achieved or the angles accurately measured.

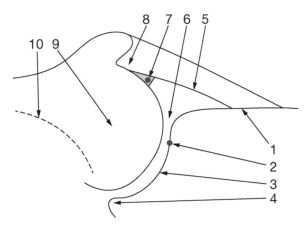

Figure 13.24 Diagram of a coronal section of the infant hip to show the anatomical landmarks; the curvature of the acetabulum is exaggerated on this diagram to demonstrate the landmarks better.

(1) The iliac wing
(2) the bony rim or turning point. This is the point at which the curvature of the bone changes from concave to convex. It is the most lateral point of the concave bony socket
(3) the bony roof of the acetabulum; this is a broad area, not a single point
(4) the lower limb of the bony acetabulum (os ileum)
(5) the joint capsule
(6) the cartilaginous roof of the acetabulum
(7) the centre of the acetabular labrum, defined as the point of the strongest echo
(8) the synovial fold
(9) the femoral head
(10) the chondro-osseus border. The appearance of the chondro-osseus border is dependent on the stage of development (ossification) and the section taken in the ultrasound image

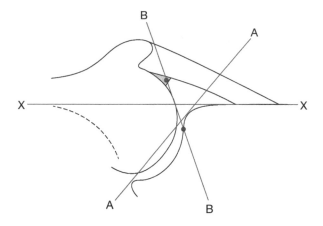

Figure 13.25 The same diagram, showing the connecting lines used for calculation of the angles in the classification of developmental dysplasia.

The three lines are:
- The base line, marked X to X; this is drawn along the iliac wing;
- The bony roof line, marked A to A. This is drawn from the lower limb of the ilium (point 4 in **Figure 13.24**) and is a tangent touching the bony roof of the acetabulum; and
- The cartilaginous roof line, marked B to B. This is drawn from the bony rim or turning point (point 2 in **Figure 13.24**) to pass through the centre of the acetabular labrum (point 7 in **Figure 13.24**). Previous literature used the tip of the labrum, but it was not always possible to identify that precise point.

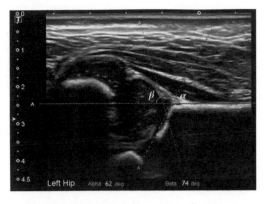

Figure 13.26 A Graf type 1 hip, with lines superimposed for α and β angle measurements.

The Graf classification system uses these three lines superimposed on the image to measure the key angles; dedicated software enables the sonographer to electronically superimpose the standard lines on the image as shown in **Figure 13.26** so that the angles are calculated automatically.

The three lines do not normally intersect at a common point; this would be the case only if the bony rim was angular, in other words with a very sharp change from concavity to convexity in the bony socket. If all three lines were to converge at one point, it is more than likely that the bony rim has been wrongly identified.[13]

The angles created by the intersections of these lines are used to evaluate the alignment of the structures forming the hip joint in the Graf classification of hip development or dysplasia. In a dislocated hip, angles cannot be measured.

The α **(alpha) angle**, or bony roof angle, is that formed by the intersection of the baseline with the bony roof line. The alpha angle gives the depth of the acetabulum, to enable evaluation of the size of the bony socket. The normal value is equal to or greater than 60°; less than 60° suggests dysplasia of the acetabulum, although this does depend on age as well. A shallow acetabulum in a baby less than 12 weeks old (the age should be adjusted for premature babies) may be due to physiological immaturity, but if found after 12 weeks of age it signifies dysplasia.[14] However, all babies with abnormal findings on ultrasound should be reviewed clinically.[11]

The β **(beta) angle**, or cartilaginous roof angle, is that formed by the intersection of the baseline with the cartilaginous roof line. The beta angle evaluates the size of the cartilaginous roof and is useful in classifying the degree of dysplasia. Beta angles should be assessed only with the hip at rest. 'There is considerable variability in the measurement of this angle and it is, therefore, not always used'.[14]

Type 1 hips have alpha angles of 60° or over. These are mature hips with a normal deep acetabulum and a centred femoral head (**Figure 13.27**).

α angle	β angle	Classification
60 or over	<55	1
50–59	55–77	2a (0–12 weeks)
50–59	55–77	2b (>12 weeks)
43–49	<77	2c
43–49	>77	D
<43		3 or 4

Figure 13.27 A table of the α (alpha) and β (beta) angles with the Graf classification progressing from type 1 (normal) to type 4.

Type 2a are those under 3 months of age with a shallow acetabulum and alpha angles of 50–59°. These are considered to be physiologically immature hips but stable. A rescan is needed to assess further at 12 weeks of age. Type 2b are the infants of over 3 months who have shallow acetabulae with alpha angles of between 50 and 59°, also considered by Graf to be inherently stable.

The most important group for the sonographer to identify is type 2c with shallow acetabulae and angles of 43–49°. These are considered to be unstable and require immediate treatment.

Type D are hips that are decentring or about to decentre and types 3 and 4 are completely decentred, or dislocated, although this is not a term used by Graf.

Figures 13.28, **13.29** and **13.30** demonstrate the line placement and angle measurements. The baby scanned in **Figure 13.30** was 4 months old. Both femoral heads are decentred and, in both hips the bony roof is poor, the bony rim is flattened and the cartilage is displaced downwards. As the alpha angle measures less than 43°, these are both classified as Graf type 4: severely dysplastic hips.

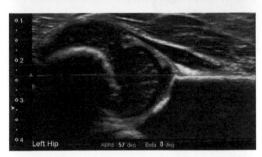

Figure 13.28 A normal left hip. The femoral head can be seen to be clearly centred within the acetabulum, the lines are correctly placed and there is an α (alpha) angle of 65°. This was classified as a Graf type 1: a normally developed hip joint.

Figure 13.29 The α (alpha) angle is 57° and, as this was a baby of less than 12 weeks old, the hip was classified as type 2a, being immature rather than dysplastic. If this were the appearance in a baby of 12 weeks or older, the hip would be regarded as dysplastic.

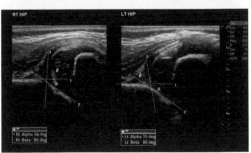

Figure 13.30 The right alpha angle is 34° and the beta angle is 86°. The left alpha angle is 35° and the beta angle is 80°.

The initial treatment recommended for severely dysplastic hips is to place the baby in an abduction orthosis such as a Pavlik harness, which holds the legs in abduction to maintain the position of the femoral head within the acetabulum and encourage normal development (**Figure 13.32**). Follow-up scans are performed at intervals during this treatment to assess the change in the alpha angle in order to monitor the position and the stability of the femoral head within the acetabulum.

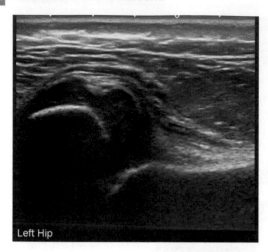

Figure 13.31 Hip with an unmeasurable alpha angle; it has not been possible to place the lines and measure the angles, because the femoral head is decentred. This was classified as a Graf type 4 hip.

Left Hip

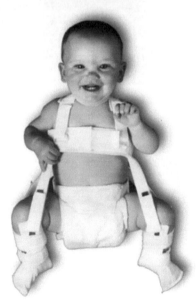

Figure 13.32 A child in a Pavlik harness, which holds the femoral heads within the acetabulae.

Although infant hip images are often viewed as per the classic sonographic orientation, with the patient's head to the left of the screen, it should be noted that Graf, the originator of this technique, asserts that image orientation with the baby's head to the top of the screen, similar to a pelvic radiographic projection, is the easiest for our brain to interpret.[13] The monitors on many machines are incompatible with a sideways-oriented display, and Graf suggests that orientation with the baby's head towards the right is the next best way. This is why the images in **Figures 13.26**, **13.28**, **13.29** and **13.31** have been taken with the head to the right, whereas those in **Figure 13.30** are conventionally oriented. Both hips are always scanned in the same orientation (as in **Figure 13.30**), and only the correct labelling will enable them to be identified.

THE KNEE

Although MRI is probably the most sensitive, specific and accurate non-invasive method in the evaluation of the knee, sonography plays an important role in imaging this joint, particularly in the study of the extensor mechanism, collateral ligaments and popliteal space.[15] Ultrasound is a portable, accessible and low-cost method compared with MRI, and permits an easy dynamic examination. It is invaluable in sports medicine, and is undoubtedly the preferred imaging modality to study soft-tissue lesions dynamically.[16]

Indications

Typically, the evaluation of the knee is focused on one anatomical area based on the clinical findings. The indications for ultrasound of the knee mainly include soft-tissue injury, tendon and collateral ligament pathology, soft-tissue masses or swelling and effusion. Ultrasound should be the first imaging method for the following presentations:

- Localised stiffness, pain or swelling noted over medial or lateral aspects.
- Localised point tenderness over the insertion site of the quadriceps or patellar tendons.

- Suspicion of partial or total tendon or ligament tears.
- Suspicion of Baker's cyst.

Patient preparation

The lower limb should be uncovered to allow an easy positioning of the structures. A clean blanket for warmth and privacy should cover the pelvic region. Careful communication ensures that the patient not only understands what to do, but also why it has to be done.

Imaging procedure

The knee should be examined using a linear array transducer of at least 7.5 MHz frequency.

Initially, the patient should sit, or lie supine, with 20–30° of flexion at the knee. This may be achieved by placing a small pillow beneath the popliteal space if required.

The anterior knee evaluation starts in a long axis plane, with the probe placed in the midline, immediately superior to the patella (**Figure 13.33**). This enables examination of the quadriceps tendon, suprapatellar fat pad, suprapatellar synovial recess and, immediately superficial to the femur, the pre-femoral fat pad.

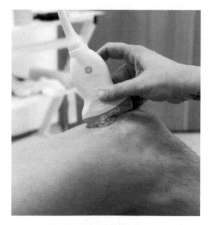 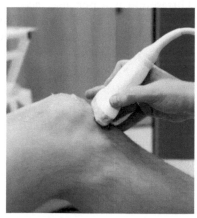

Figure 13.33 Position for a suprapatellar scan in the longitudinal plane.

Figure 13.34 Position for a transverse scan of the patellar tendon.

Still in a long axis, the probe may be moved distally to the patella, to examine the patellar tendon from its origin down to its distal insertion. Deep to the patellar tendon, the infrapatellar fat pad (Hoffa's fat pad) can be seen.

Transverse scans should also be performed (**Figure 13.34**), as well as dynamic evaluation. The classic description of the quadriceps tendon is of a trilaminar appearance, with rectus femoris most anteriorly, vastus medialis and lateralis as the middle layer and vastus intermedius as the deepest layer, but recent research has suggested that there may be more layers and as many as six tendons with variable fusion points, so very careful observation is required in cases of patellar instability.[17]

The medial collateral ligament prevents medial widening of the joint space and is stiff with the knee in extension, so the leg is externally rotated, keeping the knee flexed, and the probe is placed at the long axis of the medial collateral ligament, in an oblique orientation, to enable examination of the ligament from the medial femoral condyle to the proximal tibial metaphysis. Dynamic assessment of the ligament integrity can be performed.[18]

The leg is next internally rotated and the lower edge of the probe placed on the head of the fibula to locate the lateral collateral ligament, a complex structure that stabilises the knee against valgus stress and internal rotation. The ligament is scanned from the lateral aspect of the fibular head to the lateral femoral condyle.

To image the posterior aspect of the knee, the patient is turned to the prone position, and the probe is placed over the knee joint and rotated to visualise both transverse and longitudinal sections (**Figure 13.35**).

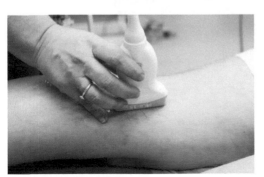

Figure 13.35 Scan position of the posterior aspect of the knee joint, with the patient lying prone.

If cruciate ligament lesions are suspected, based on clinical findings and positive clinical tests, MRI should be performed. Nevertheless, ultrasound can provide indirect signs for the assessment of the cruciate ligaments, such as fluid collections and dynamic assessment of the degree of tibial subluxation during stress manoeuvres.[18]

Image analysis

The patellar tendon is seen as a hyperechoic, fibrillar and uniform structure, with a thin elliptical cross-sectional area extending from the anterior/inferior surface of the patella down to the tibial anterior tuberosity (**Figure 13.36**). The long tendon fibres can be distinguished. Prepatellar bursitis is demonstrated on **Figure 13.37** as an anechoic area on the image, superficial to the patellar tendon.

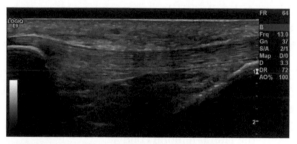

Figure 13.36 The normal patellar tendon.

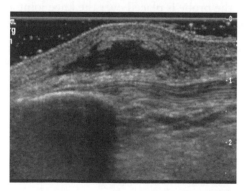

Figure 13.37 Prepatellar bursitis.

The collateral ligaments can be appreciated as hyperechoic structures with a fibrillar pattern (**Figure 13.38**). If thickening and hypoechoic changes are observed in the lateral collateral ligament, a close inspection of the medial meniscus should be performed. If meniscal tears are suspected, the patient should be referred for an MRI examination, since it is the most accurate method for diagnosing meniscal tears.

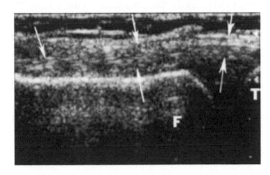

Figure 13.38 The medial collateral ligament, showing normal appearances.

A Baker's cyst is the most common bursal finding in sonography and may be seen on scanning the posterior aspect of the knee and upper calf. It appears as a well-defined fluid collection between the semimembranosus tendon medially and the medial head of gastrocnemius laterally, resulting from distension of the semimembranosus gastrocnemius bursa (**Figure 13.39**). This bursa communicates with the knee joint and the fluid in the bursa surrounds the medial gastrocnemius tendon in a C shape. It should be evaluated in longitudinal section to determine its extent and to assess for rupture.[19]

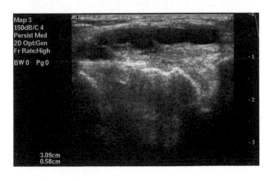

Figure 13.39 A Baker's cyst at the posterior aspect of the left knee.

THE ANKLE AND FOOT

Indications

Sonography of the ankle and foot is highly useful for examination of the superficial structures, particularly the tendons, which may be examined for tenosynovitis and other tendinopathies such as tendinosis, tears or longitudinal splits. Ultrasound may also demonstrate joint abnormalities, a ganglion, cyst, haematoma, plantar fasciitis, bursitis and Morton's neuroma.

Dynamic assessment of possible subluxation and for tarsal tunnel compression can be undertaken with ultrasound.

Sonography may also be used for injection guidance and to check for postoperative integrity.

Patient preparation

Although no physical preparation is needed, a careful history should be taken to consider systemic joint disease, sporting or occupational activities, as well as local trauma. Examinations of the foot in particular are often focused on a specific clinical question.

Imaging procedure

A small-footprint, high-frequency transducer (at least 10 MHz) is recommended. As is often the case, colourflow and power Doppler may be used for detecting the degree of vascularity within structures. The examination position will vary with the specific anatomy under investigation and so will be described individually for each of the four aspects of the ankle: anterior, medial, lateral and posterior.[6] Scanning of each part is undertaken in both longitudinal and transverse sections. Ease of access and patient flexibility may facilitate comparison between each side. Care must be taken to angle the probe continuously during movement around the ankle so that the beam remains perpendicular to the tendons in order to avoid anisotropy, an artefact illustrated and described in more detail in this chapter in the section on 'The shoulder'.

For the **anterior** aspect of the ankle, the patient should be seated or lying on the couch with the knee flexed at 45° so that the plantar surface of the foot is flat on the couch (**Figure 13.40**). This enables examination of the anterior tibio-talar joint recess for effusion, loose bodies and synovial thickening, and the tendons of tibialis anterior, extensor hallucis longus, extensor digitorum longus and, when present, the peroneus tertius tendon. It may also be possible to see the inferior tibio-fibular ligament by scanning superior and medial to the lateral malleolus in an oblique plane over the distal tibia and fibula.

For the **medial** aspect of the ankle, the seated patient externally rotates the leg, or the supine patient turns sideways into the lateral decubitus position, lying on the affected side. The transducer is placed proximal to the medial malleolus, over the tibialis posterior and the flexor digitorum longus tendons, which can be scanned transversely from the myotendinous junction to their different insertions. The flexor hallucis longus tendon may also be seen posteriorly, medial to the Achilles tendon. The tibial nerve can be identified at the level of the malleolus, between the flexor digitorum tendon anteriorly and the flexor hallucis longus tendon posteriorly. The nerve can then be traced proximally and distally.

For the **lateral** aspect of the ankle, the patient is again in the lateral decubitus position, but with the affected side uppermost (**Figure 13.41**). The transducer is placed proximal to the lateral malleolus and the peroneal tendons identified in transverse section. The peroneus longus tendon can be followed from the myotendinous junction distally to its insertion at the base of the first metatarsal and medial cuneiform; the more distal portion may be more easily scanned if the leg is internally rotated to bring the plantar region of the foot uppermost. The peroneus brevis tendon can be followed to the base of the fifth metatarsal. For both of these tendons, rotation of the ankle and dorsiflexion of the foot during scanning may assist in demonstrating any subluxation.[20] It may also be possible to see the anterior talo-fibular, calcaneo-fibular and anterior tibio-fibular ligaments using oblique angulation of the probe.

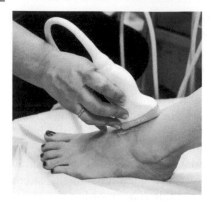

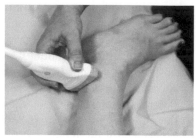

Figure 13.40 Positioning for scanning the anterior aspect of the ankle joint; the plantar aspect of the foot is flat on the couch.

Figure 13.41 Scanning the lateral aspect of the ankle joint and peroneal tendons

For the **posterior** structures of the ankle, the patient should lie in the prone position, with the feet overhanging the end of the couch (**Figure 13.42**). The Achilles tendon can then be examined in longitudinal and transverse sections from the myotendinous junctions of the medial and lateral heads of the gastrocnemius and soleus muscles to its calcaneal insertion. Plantar- and dorsiflexion while scanning may assist in the evaluation of rupture. The transducer is tilted in the transverse axis on each side to assess the peritendinous envelope. In the longitudinal plane, the transducer should be placed over the plantar aspect of the hindfoot to examine the calcaneal insertion.

The **plantar aspect of the foot** may be examined during the position for the medial and posterior aspects of the ankle as described previously, or the patient may be seated on the couch with the legs extended so that the soles of the feet are vertical to the couch (**Figure 13.43**). The plantar fascia can be scanned in both long- and short-axis planes from its proximal origin on the medial calcaneal tubercle to its distal division where it merges into the soft tissues. To examine the interphalangeal or interdigital spaces, the probe should be placed longitudinally on the plantar aspect of the first interdigital space while the sonographer applies pressure on the dorsal surface. The transducer is moved laterally, with its centre at the level of the metatarsal heads, and the process repeated for the remaining interspaces and then again in the transverse plane. If a Morton's neuroma is suspected, pressure can be applied to reproduce the patient's symptoms; this requires good communication. The intermetatarsal bursa lies on the dorsal aspect of the interdigital nerve, and care must be taken to correctly identify a neuroma and differentiate it from the bursa.[21] If there is suspected inflammatory arthritis, the metatarsophalangeal joints should be examined in this position as well as dorsally for effusion, synovial hypertrophy, vascularity and bony erosions.

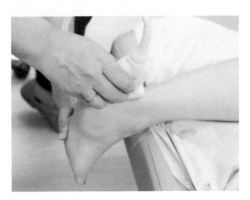

Figure 13.42 (left) Scanning the Achilles tendon.

Figure 13.43 (right) Scanning the plantar aspect of the foot to check for Morton's neuroma.

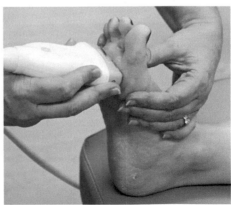

Image analysis

The sonographer has applied a special image reconstruction technique to give an extended field of view in **Figure 13.44**. This is the normal side, imaged for comparison with the injured side in **Figure 13.45**. Comparison of the images enables identification not just of the Achilles tear but also of the disruption and the considerable soft-tissue inflammation in the region of the tear.

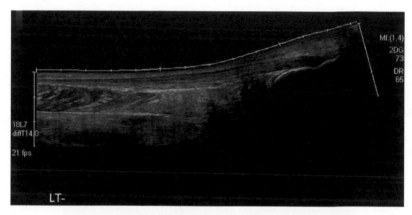

Figure 13.44 Normal left (LT) Achilles tendon.

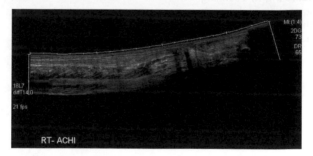

Figure 13.45 This is the same patient as examined in **Figure 13.44**, but the right (RT) Achilles tendon has a full-thickness tear, seen in the very near field.

A Morton's neuroma is demonstrated in **Figures 13.46** and **13.47**. This is a relatively common, benign but painful condition. The white arcs are the metatarsals, as numbered, so this is in the third intertarsal space. The measurement callipers show this to be approximately 2 cm in diameter.

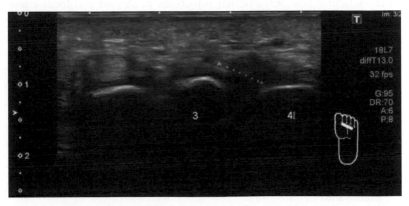

Figure 13.46 A scan of the plantar aspect of the foot in transverse section, showing a Morton's neuroma (between the callipers).

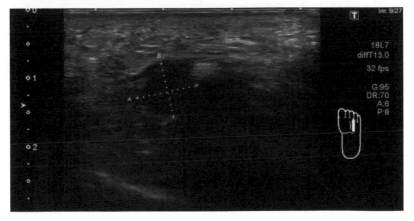

Figure 13.47 The same Morton's neuroma in longitudinal section.

ULTRASOUND-GUIDED INTERVENTIONS

Intra-articular and periarticular injections of steroid and local anaesthetic are commonly administered for relief of pain or inflammation and have historically been performed 'blind' using palpation of anatomical landmarks, with varied clinical outcomes.[22]

With the growing availability and affordability of ultrasound systems, ultrasound-guided steroid injections have grown in popularity in recent years, ensuring better results by:

- enabling visualisation of anatomy which may be difficult to locate due factors such as a high BMI (body mass index) or pathology, so helping with accurate needle placement, including placement into deep, impalpable or difficult areas such as the hip or tarsal joints;
- ensuring that tendons, vessels and nerves are avoided during needle placement;
- enabling absolute accuracy of needle placement, so that, if there is no symptomatic improvement, this eradicates the possibility that the injection was in the wrong place.

Indications

Steroid injections can be performed for a number of reasons, including:

- to relieve pain in order to facilitate rehabilitation exercises;
- to relieve pain if treatments such as rehabilitation and other medication have been unsuccessful;
- as temporary pain relief in patients awaiting surgery;
- as a pain-relieving measure in patients who are not surgical candidates;
- to relieve joint inflammation in diseases such as rheumatoid arthritis.

Intra-articular and periarticular pain can be caused by a myriad of conditions. Some are generic and can affect any joint, such as inflammatory arthritis. Some are specific to the processes within a particular joint or region, for example:

- **Shoulder**: pain commonly caused by the process of impingement – injection to the subacromial bursa.
- **Elbow**: pain commonly caused by 'tennis' or 'golfer's' elbow – injection into the common extensor or flexor origins, respectively.
- **Wrist**: pain commonly caused by de Quervain's tenosynovitis – injection into the tendon sheath of the first extensor tendon.
- **Hip**: pain commonly caused by trochanteric bursitis – injection into the region of the trochanteric bursa.

Patient preparation

No physical patient preparation is needed but consent and checks for contraindications are vital.

Valid, informed consent is crucial and should include:

- an explanation of the nature of the condition;
- details of the treatment and the nature of the drugs to be used;
- possible risks and side effects and the likely efficacy and benefits;
- implications of not having the procedure.

A combination of corticosteroid and local anaesthetic is administered. Each drug has known side effects and contraindications. Most departments have their own cautions and contraindications depending on local protocols; obvious and universal contraindications would include allergy to any of the drugs, or current local and systemic infections.

Whether this should be a sterile or aseptic technique again depends on local guidelines, which vary from advising a sterile technique incorporating the use of sterile probe cover, to a simple aseptic technique. Sterile ultrasound gel should be used in all interventional cases.[23]

Imaging procedure

It is becoming increasingly popular in rheumatology departments, having made the decision to inject clinically, that ultrasound guidance is used purely to direct the steroid into the appropriate target. In an imaging department, an injection is usually performed following a diagnostic scan where a decision is made, based on scan findings, that an injection would be useful. The success of a guided injection relies heavily on the operator's ability to do the following:

- Set up the ultrasound equipment to give optimum visualisation of the point of interest. This requires understanding of the physics of ultrasound and the functions of the ultrasound controls.
- Recognise the anatomy to be injected and the anatomy to be avoided. As well as greyscale imaging, colourflow and power Doppler are employed to ensure avoidance of any vascular structures during needle placement.
- Have excellent hand–eye coordination in order to accurately and efficiently guide the needle into place.

Accurate and safe needle placement requires the operator to be able to visualise the needle from the point of skin puncture to when it reaches the target and ideally to maintain visualisation during the administration of the drugs to ensure that they infiltrate appropriately. A high-frequency linear array probe is used.

Image analysis

In this case (**Figure 13.48**), an aseptic technique is used, which is more usual in practice than a full sterile procedure. A needle guide is not being used and again this is the more usual procedure, because, for optimum visualisation of the needle, it should be as close to parallel to the skin surface as possible in order to generate a specular reflection of the ultrasound beam.

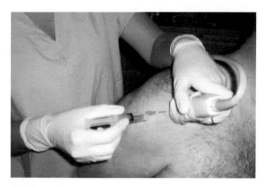

Figure 13.48 The patient is positioned seated on a stool for a subacromial bursa injection in the shoulder, while the sonographer performs the procedure from a standing position behind the patient.

A good example of specular reflection from the length of the needle is demonstrated in **Figure 13.49**. This is easy to achieve in smaller, superficial structures, but harder in deeper regions such as the trochanteric bursa of the hip, or the subacromial bursa of the shoulder, where a steeper angle is necessary and therefore specular reflection is compromised. Hand–eye coordination is crucial to maintain needle visualisation throughout.

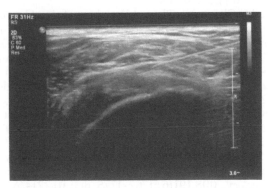

Figure 13.49 The needle can be seen clearly, traversing the deltoid muscle and entering the subacromial bursa.

Ultrasound-guided aspirations

When performing an ultrasound-guided aspiration, exactly the same principles are employed as for guided steroid injections, but, rather than administering drugs when the needle is in place, fluid is instead removed.

As in the case of steroid injections, prior to the widespread use of ultrasound, joint or bursal aspirations were also performed 'blind', again with varying degrees of success.[24] Utilising ultrasound confirms the diagnosis of an effusion within a swollen, painful joint and also identifies complications such as loculation or synovial proliferation within the effusion.

It is clinically beneficial to aspirate the maximum amount of fluid from an affected joint and the use of ultrasound has been shown to be superior to 'blind' aspiration. Sibbitt et al.[25] found a huge difference in quantity of fluid aspirated when using ultrasound guidance, in comparison with a blind technique.

REFERENCES

1. Largacha M, Parsons IM 4th, Campbell B, Titelman RM, Smith KL, Matsen F 3rd. Deficits in shoulder function and general health associated with sixteen common shoulder diagnoses: A study of 2674 patients. *Journal of Shoulder and Elbow Surgery* 2006;**15**(1):30–39. doi: 10.1016/j.jse.2005.04.006.

2. Pribicevic M. Chapter 7: The epidemiology of shoulder pain: A narrative review of the literature. In: Ghosh S, (ed.), *Pain in perspective*. London: IntechOpen, 2012:147–186. doi: 10.5772/52931.

3. Lin C-W, Chen Y-H, Chen W-S. Application of ultrasound and ultrasound-guided intervention for evaluating elbow joint pathologies. *Journal of Medical Ultrasound* 2012;**20**(2):87–95. doi: 10.1016/j.jmu.2012.04.007.

4. Middleton WD, Teefey SA, Boyer MI. Hand and wrist sonography. *Ultrasound Quarterly* 2001;**17**(1):21–36. doi: 10.1097/00013644-200103000-00004.

5. Bianchi S, Della Santa D, Glauser T, Beaulieu JY, van Aaken J. Sonography of masses of the wrist and hand. *American Journal of Roentgenology* 2008;**191**(6):1767–1775. doi: 10.2214/AJR.07.4003.

6. AIUM (American Institute of Ultrasound in Medicine). *AIUM practice parameter for the performance of a musculoskeletal ultrasound examination*. Laurel, MD: AIUM, 2017:1–25. Available at: https://www.aium.org/resources/guidelines/musculoskeletal.pdf.

7. Tagliafico A, Rubino M, Autuori A, Bianchi S, Martinoli C. Wrist and hand ultrasound. *Seminar Musculoskeletal Radiology* 2007;**11**(2):95–104. doi: 10.1055/s-2007-1001875.

8. Teefey SA, Middleton WD, Boyer MI. Sonography of the hand and wrist. *Seminars in Ultrasound, CT, and MRI* 2000;**21**(3):192–204. doi: 10.1016/s0887-2171(00)90042-8.

9. Sewell MD, Rosendahl K, Eastwood DM. Developmental dysplasia of the hip. *British Medical Journal* 2009;**339**:b4454. doi: 10.1136/bmj.b4454.

10. NICE (National Institute for Health and Care Excellence). *Postnatal care up to 8 weeks after birth. Clinical guideline [CG37]*, 2015. Available at: https://www.nice.org.uk/guidance/cg37/chapter/1-Recommendations#maintaining-infant-health.

11. PHE (Public Health England). *Guidance. Newborn and infant physical examination (NIPE) screening programme handbook*, 2021. Available at: https://www.gov.uk/government/publications/newborn-and-

infant-physical-examination-programme-handbook/newborn-and-infant-physical-examination-screening-programme-handbook#examination-of-the-hips.

12. Graf R. *Hip sonography: Diagnosis and management of infant hip dysplasia*, 2nd edn. Heidelberg: Springer-Verlag, 2006.

13. Graf R. *Essentials of infant hip sonography*. Stolzalpe: Stolzalpe Sonocentre, 2014.

14. SoR (Society of Radiographers) & BMUS (British Medical Ultrasound Society). *Guidelines for professional ultrasound practice*. SCoR and BMUS, 2021. Available at: https://www.sor.org/learning-advice/professional-body-guidance-and-publications/documents-and-publications/policy-guidance-document-library.

15. Grobbelaar N, Bouffard JA. Sonography of the knee, a pictorial review. *Seminars in Ultrasound, CT MRI* 2000;21(3):231–274. doi: 10.1016/S0887-2171(00)90045-3.

16. Chiang Y-P, Wang T-G, Hsieh S-F. Application of ultrasound in sports Injury. *Journal of Medical Ultrasound* 2013;21(1):1–8. doi: 10.1016/j.jmu.2013.01.008.

17. Grob K, Manestar M, Filgueira L, Ackland T, Gilbey H, Kuster MS. New insight in the architecture of the quadriceps tendon. *Journal of Experimental Orthopaedics* 2016;3(1):32. doi: 10.1186/s40634-016-0068-y.

18. Sekiya JK, Swaringen JC, Wojtys EM, Jacobson JA. Diagnostic ultrasound evaluation of posterolateral corner knee injuries. *Arthroscopy* 2010:26(4):494–499. doi: 10.1016/j.arthro.2009.08.023.

19. Ward EE, Jacobson JA, Fessell DP, Hayes CW, van Holsbeeck M. Sonographic detection of Baker's cysts: Comparison with MR imaging. *American Journal of Roentgenology* 2001;176(2):373–380. doi: 10.2214/ajr.176.2.1760373.

20. Bianchi S, Martinoli C, Gaignot C, De Gautard R, Meyer JM. Ultrasound of the ankle: Anatomy of the tendons, bursae, and ligaments. *Seminar Musculoskeletal Radiology* 2005;9(3):243–259. doi: 10.1055/s-2005-921943.

21. Fessell DP, Jacobson JA. Ultrasound of the hindfoot and midfoot. *Radiologic Clinics of North America* 2008;46(6):1027–1043. doi: 10.1016/j.rcl.2008.08.006.

22. Raza K, Lee CY, Pilling D, Heaton S, Situnayake RD, Carruthers DM, et al. Ultrasound guidance allows accurate needle placement and aspiration from small joints in patients with early inflammatory arthritis. *Rheumatology* 2003;42(8):976–979. doi: 10.1093/rheumatology/keg269.

23. UKHSA (UK Health Security Agency). *Guidance. Good infection prevention practice: Using ultrasound gel*, 2022. Available at: https://www.gov.uk/government/publications/ultrasound-gel-good-infection-prevention-practice/good-infection-prevention-practice-using-ultrasound-gel.
24. Balint PV, Kane D, Hunter J, McInnes IB, Field M, Sturrock RD. Ultrasound guided versus conventional joint and soft tissue fluid aspiration in rheumatology practice: A pilot study. *The Journal of Rheumatology* 2002;**29**(10):2209–2213. PMID: 12375335.
25. Sibbitt WL Jr, Peisajovich A, Michael AA, Park KS, Sibbitt RR, Band PA, et al. Does sonographic needle guidance affect the clinical outcome of intra-articular injections? *The Journal of Rheumatology* 2009;**36**(9):1892–1902. doi: 10.3899/jrheum.090013.

CHAPTER 14

EMERGENCY AND INTERVENTIONAL ULTRASOUND

Emergency ultrasound: FAST   322
Interventional ultrasound   330
References   335

EMERGENCY ULTRASOUND: FAST

For many years, it has been acknowledged that physical evaluation of the trauma patient is unreliable, even in expert hands. Cardiac tamponade (accumulation of fluid, blood or other substances in the pericardial space) and massive intraperitoneal haemorrhage can be fatal if not diagnosed and treated quickly; therefore, a tool to diagnose these conditions is vital. In the 1970s Grace Rozycki, an American trauma surgeon, developed an ultrasound technique focused primarily on the detection of intra-abdominal bleeding rather than on abdominal organ injury.[1] This has become known as focused assessment with sonography in trauma, or FAST.

The basis of FAST is to detect fluid in any of the dependent sites of the body where it might collect: the perihepatic and perisplenic areas, the pericardium and the pelvis. Various protocol extensions have been proposed, with 'eFAST' or extended FAST, including interrogation of the lung fields, being regarded as one of the most practical and time-efficient add-ons, with sensitivity in trauma patients better than that of supine chest radiography.[2] Sonography of the lung fields is more fully described in Chapter 11 on 'The respiratory system – lungs'.

Point-of-care or emergency medicine ultrasound has developed as a safe, rapid imaging technique, with a mean FAST examination time of between 3 and 4 minutes.[3] Ultrasound is non-invasive, easily repeatable and does not need contrast media or any special patient preparation. Although FAST does not yield the organ detail of computed tomography (CT) scanning, studies have reported that, for detection of intra-abdominal injuries, a sensitivity of 86% with specificity of 98% and accuracy of 98% can be achieved.[4]

Unlike formal ultrasound, FAST can be performed by specialist operators who have had limited training in ultrasound but have become competent in this specific area. The equipment used is small and easily transportable, therefore FAST can be performed as soon as a first responder is in contact with the patient. This may be while in an ambulance or air ambulance, and FAST has even been trialled on board the International Space Station.[5] It is important that anyone using focused ultrasound is trained to scan and interpret the findings, and that their work is audited to ensure continuing competency, in the same way that any other ultrasound practice should be.

Indications

FAST should be performed on all patients presenting with an acute history of blunt abdominal trauma or cardiac tamponade, and to check for haemoperitoneum or haemopericardium where internal bleeding is suspected.

Contraindications

Even in the emergency situation, there are possible contraindications to ultrasound, including:

- if the patient has a more pressing problem such as obstructed airway or cardiac arrest;
- if there are external injuries that prevent scanning directly on the skin, for example burns;
- if there is a clear indication for emergency laparotomy.

Patient preparation

The person performing the scan should wash their hands before and after the scan or wear non-latex medical examination gloves.

No specific patient preparation is required, although the **pelvis should be imaged prior to any catheterisation** in order to use the full bladder as an acoustic window. Access points are exposed and acoustic gel is applied directly to the skin. Sterile gel should be used if the skin is broken or if interventional procedures are likely to follow.[6]

Imaging procedure

The probe should be an appropriate shape to scan between the ribs and other places of limited access: a tight-radius sector scanner is ideal; however, a regular curvilinear probe will suffice if that is the only one available. A low frequency (3–5 MHz) should be used to allow adequate penetration for the deep structures; detailed resolution is not a priority in trauma. The focus and the depth should be set according to the patient's build. Ideally, the equipment will have a default setting for FAST scanning.

The FAST examination is best performed with the patient supine, their arms slightly abducted to allow access. The patient may be unable to cooperate but, if conscious, may be able to aid the examination by taking a deep inspiration to bring the diaphragm and the upper abdominal organs downwards below the lower costal margin.

There are four basic views (perihepatic, perisplenic, pericardial and pelvic) to interrogate the main areas where fluid may collect.[7] Each of these four areas is scanned in turn. If there is a positive finding in any of these areas, the result is a positive FAST scan.

The perihepatic view is shown in **Figure 14.1**. The probe is placed in the coronal section in the right upper quadrant, where the right costal margin meets the midaxillary line. Side-to-side movements, using the liver as an acoustic window, allow a clear view of Morrison's pouch, incorporating the diaphragm, liver and right kidney. There should be no free fluid between the liver and diaphragm, or between the liver and the kidney.

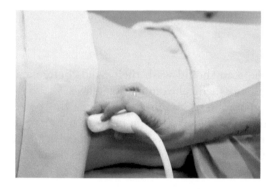

Figure 14.1 Positioning for the perihepatic view.

The probe is placed in the coronal section in the left upper quadrant where the left costal margin meets the mid-axillary line, but slightly higher than on the right, ideally between the 9th and 11th ribs to obtain the perisplenic view (**Figure 14.2**). The probe is moved from side to side to obtain a clear view of the spleen and, using this organ as an acoustic window, the diaphragm and the left kidney are also imaged. There should be no free fluid anywhere around the spleen.

For the pericardial view, the probe is laid almost flat on the patient's epigastrium and angled cephalad and slightly towards the left shoulder

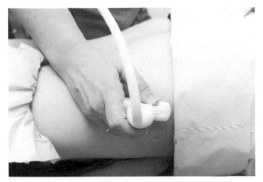

Figure 14.2 Positioning for the perisplenic view.

(**Figure 14.3**). Enough pressure is required to indent the epigastrium below the xiphisternum. The correct angulation will demonstrate the four chambers of the heart. The four chambers of the heart with cardiac pulsation should be clearly seen. Any free fluid generally appears as a dark stripe in the pericardium around the left ventricle. A small amount of free fluid is commonly seen in older patients with cardiac problems; this should be taken into account when undertaking FAST.

For the pelvic view, the probe is placed just above the symphysis pubis and angled caudally until an image of the bladder and pelvic

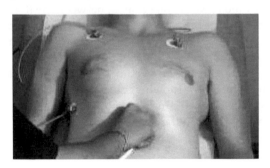

Figure 14.3 Positioning for the pericardial view.

organs is obtained, demonstrating the pouch of Douglas (recto-uterine pouch) in the female patient or recto-vesical pouch in the male patient (**Figure 14.4**). If required, a transverse view can be used by rotating the probe through 90° and again angling caudally. The urinary bladder is easily demonstrated if full, and there should be no free fluid posterior to the bladder. However, if there is significant bleeding, bowel may be seen floating in the fluid. Peristalsis will distinguish intraluminal fluid from free fluid. A small amount of fluid can sometimes be seen in the pouch of Douglas post-ovulation or post-menstruation; this should be taken into account in women of menstrual age.

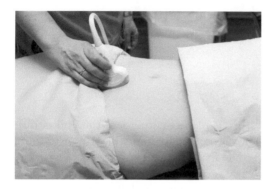

Figure 14.4 Positioning for the pelvic view.

Image analysis

Figures 14.5 and **14.6** are both taken from a FAST scan performed by an emergency clinician on an adult male who fell while cycling off-road, sustaining blunt trauma to his abdomen. **Figure 14.5** shows the perihepatic view, with free fluid in Morrison's pouch, between the liver and the right kidney. Free fluid is seen between the spleen and the left kidney in the perisplenic view (**Figure 14.6**). The spleen shows an irregular heterogeneous echotexture, in keeping with rupture.

A perisplenic view in another patient who sustained blunt abdominal trauma is demonstrated in **Figure 14.7**, showing free fluid between the spleen and diaphragm and as a pleural effusion above the diaphragm. There is some splenic damage visible in the near field.

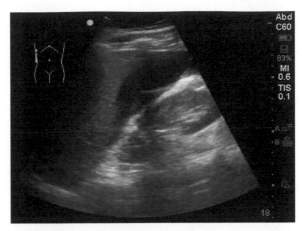

Figure 14.5 Perihepatic view following an off-road cycling accident.

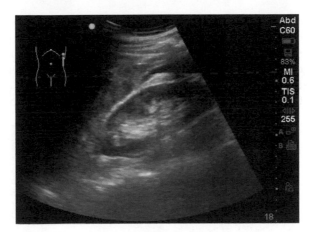

Figure 14.6 Perisplenic view; same patient as in **Figure 14.5**.

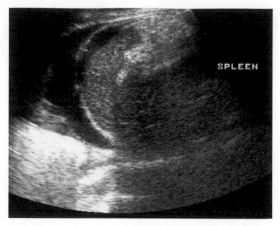

Figure 14.7 Perisplenic view of a trauma patient following a road traffic collision.

The pericardial section shown in **Figure 14.8** is best viewed in real time, to observe the four chambers of the heart with cardiac pulsation. Any free fluid generally appears as a hypoechoic (dark) band in the pericardium around the left ventricle, as in this image, where a moderate-size pericardial effusion is demonstrated (arrow). This amount of free fluid is more than would be expected due to cardiac problems.

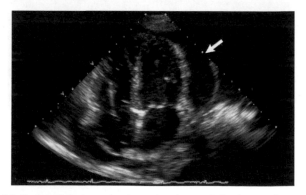

Figure 14.8 Pericardial view: the four chambers of the heart, the apex being closest to the probe at the top of the image.

Not all emergency cases are the result of trauma. **Figure 14.9** was from a FAST examination performed on a 55-year-old woman who presented to the emergency department with acute abdominal symptoms, pain and nausea. Free fluid was seen in the pelvic view and tracked to the right iliac fossa (labelled RIF FF). Where there is significant free fluid, real time sonography may demonstrate bowel floating in the fluid, and peristalsis may distinguish intraluminal fluid from free fluid. In this case, a subsequent CT scan showed omental masses, abdominal aortic pathological lymph nodes and a right adnexal mass. A biopsy sample from the omental mass showed an ovarian malignancy to be the primary tumour.

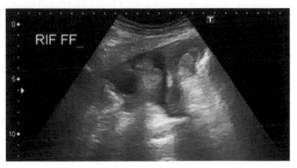

Figure 14.9 A scan of the right iliac fossa (RIF FF).

INTERVENTIONAL ULTRASOUND

Ultrasound guidance for interventional procedures is arguably better than fluoroscopy or CT because there is no radiation and better than magnetic resonance imaging (MRI) because there are no equipment/magnet issues. Other compelling advantages of ultrasound as a means to guide and perform interventions include the following:

- It is faster to set up and perform than CT biopsy.[8]
- There is a high degree of both accuracy and manoeuvrability.
- It can be performed by a small team, or even single-handed by the skilled operator, using the probe and the needle at the same time.
- Good soft-tissue imaging, with no contrast medium required, and it is possible to use Doppler to visualise vascularity.[9]
- Direct real-time visualisation of both tissue and needle movement with, for example, visual confirmation of drainages.

The technique requires practised motor skills, as well as mental conceptualisation of the three-dimensional nature inferred from a two-dimensional image plus a perspective along the line of sight of the ultrasound beam.[10] Therefore, dedicated training and continuing audit are recommended.

Indications

Ultrasound interventions and ultrasound-guided procedures include the following:

- Intracavity imaging including transoesophageal, transduodenal, transvaginal, transrectal and intravascular procedures, described within the relevant chapters.
- Insertion of drains into collections in the chest (thoracocentesis) or abdomen (paracentesis); placement of suprapubic catheters.
- Visualisation during therapeutic suction drainage of collections such as pleural effusions, ascites or other collections; percutaneous nephrostomy for kidney drainage.
- Percutaneous transhepatic or endoscopic biliary drainage after failed endoscopic retrograde cholangio-pancreatography (ERCP).[11]

- Needle placement directly into joint spaces, either for aspiration or for effective injection of pharmaceuticals such as steroids. This is particularly useful in the larger joints such as the hip or shoulder, as described in Chapter 13 'Musculoskeletal ultrasound'.
- Targeted drug delivery into joints and into lesions, including chemotherapy drugs, to increase efficacy while minimising systemic effects, as outlined in Chapter 15 'Additional technologies' in the section on 'Contrast-enhanced ultrasound (CEUS)'.
- Biopsy of solid lesions and drainage or fine-needle aspiration (FNA) of cystic lesions or fluid collections or of tissue for histological analysis in the thyroid, breast, liver, kidneys, adrenals, prostate, lymph nodes and many other organs.
- Guidance and vein compression during operative endovenous ablation therapy for varicose veins.
- Other percutaneous therapy including thermal ablation and high-intensity focused ultrasound (HIFU) of renal and liver lesions, and direct percutaneous sclerosis of vascular malformations.[12]
- Assisted reproductive procedures including hysterosalpingo-contrast sonography (HyCoSy), oocyte recovery and embryo transfer.
- Numerous obstetric and fetal medical procedures including chorionic villous sampling, amniocentesis for fluid sampling or therapeutic drainage, selective termination, membrane lasering and shunt placement for alleviation of the fluid build-up in twin-to-twin transfusion, cord sampling for blood incompatibilities, intrauterine transfusion procedures, and even in-utero fetal surgical procedures.

Patient preparation

As always, the operator should fully explain the benefits and any potential risks of the procedure to the patient (or parent or carer as appropriate) along with the alternatives, if any, in order to obtain fully informed consent. For interventional procedures, it is advisable to document this process and have it signed by the patient. Interventions require good patient cooperation for immobilisation and on occasion to coordinate breathing with needle advancement; this requires excellent communication skills.

Physical preparation would be the same as for non-interventional ultrasound of that part of the body, removing clothing or dressings to give bare skin access to a suitable acoustic window, while maintaining the patient's privacy and dignity. The patient's skin surface is cleaned before the application of sterile gel and again before needle insertion.

Coagulopathy factors must be considered along with any other possible complicating factors and contraindications.

Interventions are generally performed using a sterile technique to minimise any infection risk and dedicated probe covers are available for sonography during the procedure.

Sedation may be considered, along with the administration of local anaesthesia prior to the use of sharp instruments, depending on the type of procedure and patient preference.

Imaging procedure

All relevant prior imaging should be reviewed by the operator.

Ideally, a small footprint probe is used, to maximise the usability of the limited acoustic windows that may be available. For more superficial structures, a broadband 7.5–10 MHz transducer is recommended, whereas for deeper visualisation 3.5–5 MHz may be used. Needle guides are available but are used infrequently because they limit manoeuvrability.

An initial survey scan should be performed to identify the area of intervention and the surrounding anatomy. Once an organ or lesion has been identified, it must be imaged in two planes at right angles, with the probe visualised from directly overhead or perpendicular to the line of sight.[10] The operator should select an approach that will avoid damage to surrounding organs and vessels and can be physically maintained during the length of the procedure. The use of Doppler ultrasound enables a choice of access route avoiding major vessels.[9]

Images should be recorded that include the lesion, organ or fluid collection with identifying surrounding anatomy, and depth-to-target and other dimensions. Images taken during and after the procedure can help to demonstrate any immediate change, especially in drainages.

Dressings should be applied if required. Normal post-procedure nursing observations should be performed until the patient is stable.

Image analysis

A transjugular intrahepatic portosystemic shunt (TIPSS) procedure, which is usually performed to relieve portal hypertension by insertion of a stent to connect the portal vein directly to the hepatic vein, is demonstrated in **Figure 14.10**. In the past, fluoroscopic guidance was used for the whole procedure, but ultrasound guidance for puncture of the portal vein markedly reduces the diagnostic reference levels (DRLs) of radiation,[13] as does the use of colourflow Doppler to check the patency of the portal vein as shown here.

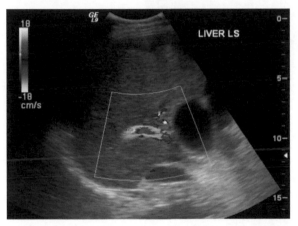

Figure 14.10 Verification of the portal vein patency following transjugular intrahepatic portosystemic shunt insertion.

Ultrasound-guided biopsies are now among the most common interventional procedures carried out in radiology departments, and include liver, renal, prostate, thyroid and breast biopsies. Biopsy is a minimally invasive way to obtain a tissue sample for histological diagnosis. **Figure 14.11** shows the liver parenchyma with the biopsy needle visible as a brighter line traversing at an angle. If the needle were to be held vertically, it would be difficult to image, because the sound needs to be reflected from it back to the transducer to produce an image. The dotted lines on the image are an electronic extension of the needle guide, as an aid to where the needle should appear. **Figure 14.12** shows an omental biopsy, utilising similar principles.

Specific interventional procedures are discussed in:

- Chapter 4 'The male reproductive system' section on 'Prostatic biopsy'.
- Chapter 5 'The gastrointestinal (GI) tract' section on 'Endoscopic ultrasound (EUS)' for pancreatic pseudocyst drainage.
- Chapter 7 'The female reproductive system' section on 'HyCoSy'.
- Chapter 13 'Musculoskeletal ultrasound' for joint interventions.

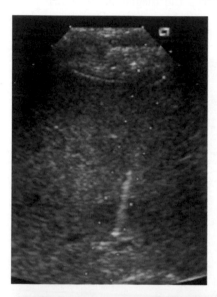

Figure 14.11 Ultrasound-guided liver biopsy.

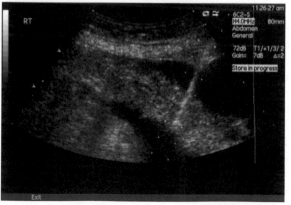

Figure 14.12 Ultrasound-guided omental biopsy.

REFERENCES

1. Rozycki GS, Shackford SR. Ultrasound, what every trauma surgeon should know. *Journal of Trauma* 1996;**40**(1):1–4. doi: 10.1097/00005373-199601000-00001.

2. Richards JR, McGahan JP. Focused assessment with sonography in trauma (FAST) in 2017: What radiologists can learn. *Radiology* 2017;**283**(1):30–48. doi: 10.1148/radiol.2017160107.

3. Brun PM, Bessereau J, Chenaitia H, Pradel AL, Deniel C, Garbaye G, et al. Stay and play eFAST or scoop and run eFAST? That is the question! *American Journal of Emergency Medicine* 2014;**32**(2):166–170. doi: 10.1016/j.ajem.2013.11.008.

4. Dolich MO, McKenney MG, Varela JE, Compton RP, McKenney KL, Cohn SM. 2,576 ultrasounds for blunt abdominal trauma. *Journal of Trauma* 2001;**50**(1):108–112. doi: 10.1097/00005373-200101000-00019.

5. Sargsyan AE, Hamilton DR, Joncs JA, Melton S, Whitson PA, Kirkpatrick AW, et al. FAST at MACH 20: Clinical ultrasound aboard the International Space Station. *Journal of Trauma* 2005;**58**(1):35–39. doi: 10.1097/01.ta.0000145083.47032.78.

6. UKHSA (UK Health Security Agency). *Guidance. Good infection prevention practice: Using ultrasound gel*, 2022. Available at: https://www.gov.uk/government/publications/ultrasound-gel-good-infection-prevention-practice/good-infection-prevention-practice-using-ultrasound-gel.

7. Brooks A, Connolly J, Chan O (eds). *Ultrasound in emergency care*. Oxford: Blackwell Publishing, 2012.

8. Winters SR, Paulson EK. Ultrasound guided biopsy: What's new? *Ultrasound Quarterly* 2005;**21**(1):19–25. PMID: 15716755.

9. Nakamoto DA, Haaga JR. Emergent ultrasound interventions. *Radiologic Clinics of North America* 2004;**42**(2):457–478. doi: 10.1016/j.rcl.2004.01.002.

10. Smith J. *AIUM practice parameter for the performance of selected ultrasound-guided procedures*. Laurel, MD: American Institute of Ultrasound in Medicine, 2014. Available at: http://www.aium.org/resources/guidelines/usguidedprocedures.pdf.

11. Baniya R, Upadhaya S, Madala S, Subedi SC, Shaik Mohammed T, Bachuwa G. Endoscopic ultrasound-guided biliary drainage versus percutaneous transhepatic biliary drainage after failed endoscopic retrograde cholangiopancreatography: A meta-analysis. *Clinical and Experimental Gastroenterology* 2017;**10**:67–74. doi: 10.2147/CEG.S132004.

12. Dogra VS, Saad WEA. *Ultrasound-guided procedures*. New York: Thieme, 2009.
13. Tavare AN, Wigham A, Hadjivassilou A, Alvi A, Papadopoulou A, Goode A, et al. Use of transabdominal ultrasound-guided transjugular portal vein puncture on radiation dose in transjugular intrahepatic portosystemic shunt formation. *Diagnostic and Interventional Radiology* 2017;**23**(3):206–210. doi: 10.5152/dir.2016.15601.

Further reading

Bowra J, McLaughlin RE. *Emergency ultrasound made easy*. London: Churchill Livingstone, 2006.

Ma OJ, Mateer J, (eds.). *Emergency ultrasound*. New York: McGraw-Hill, 2003:67–88.

RCR (Royal College of Radiologists) *Standards for providing a 24-hour interventional radiology service*, 2nd edn. London: Royal College of Radiologists, 2017:1–16. Available at: https://www.rcr.ac.uk/system/files/publication/field_publication_files/bfcr171_24hr_ir.pdf.

CHAPTER 15
ADDITIONAL TECHNOLOGIES

Contrast-enhanced ultrasound (CEUS)   338
Fusion imaging   341
Artificial intelligence (AI) in ultrasound   344
References   349

CONTRAST-ENHANCED ULTRASOUND (CEUS)

With the growth of ultrasound has come the need for an image enhancement agent to increase the information available from this modality in the same way as contrast agents are used in computed tomography (CT) and magnetic resonance imaging (MRI). The key to enhancing the returning ultrasound signal is to increase the relative echogenicity between two adjacent reflective surfaces under examination.

The criteria for a contrast medium for ultrasound are that it must:

- be sufficiently reflective to appear hyperechoic;
- be non-toxic or of low toxicity;
- have a uniform particle size;
- be able to traverse the pulmonary capillary bed in order to exit the systematic circulation;
- be stable in solution.

After many years of development, the technology universally adopted is that of encapsulated bubbles of gas that are smaller than red blood cells and are capable of circulating in the systemic vasculature. These microbubbles are now approved in more than 50 countries, and their use has opened up a new area for technological advancement in ultrasound.

The aim of using contrast agents in ultrasound imaging is to demonstrate and characterise lesions, which might otherwise be difficult to detect on B mode and Doppler ultrasound, for example isoechoic lesions that appear to be identical or of similar echotexture to the surrounding tissue or to differentiate focal liver lesions. Power Doppler can demonstrate microcirculation, but microbubble contrast agents increase the sensitivity of the examination.[1,2]

Development of ultrasound contrast agents

Commercial development of microbubbles started in the 1980s and their first use was in echocardiography. First-generation agents were stable enough to pass through the pulmonary circulation but were known to break up quickly, resulting in insufficient imaging time. The second-generation agents have been designed to increase backscatter enhancement and to last longer in the bloodstream by taking advantage of low-solubility gases such as perfluorocarbons. The shells of these bubbles are more flexible and composed of phospholipids; sometimes proteins and polymers are used. The microbubbles are self-assembling following suspension in saline and shaking. The shell material is bio-compatible and non-toxic. The gas is exhaled and the shell metabolised in the liver.

Pharmacokinetics

The pharmacokinetics of ultrasound contrast agents are different from those of the iodinated agents used in CT and the gadolinium agents used in MRI, as ultrasonic contrast agents act as pure blood pool agents and do not diffuse into the interstitial space. Contrast agents for ultrasound have a low incidence of side effects and are well tolerated by patients. They have few contraindications; they do not interact with the thyroid and are not nephrotoxic, so laboratory tests of renal function are not required before administering ultrasound contrast agents. The incidence of severe hypersensitivity or allergic events is lower than with current radiographic contrast agents, and comparable to contrast agents for MRI.[3]

Another difference is the dose. Only 2–5 ml of ultrasound contrast agent is required, in part because the microbubble detection methods are very sensitive, whereas 25 ml of contrast agent is typical for MRI, and hundreds of millilitres of iodinated agent may be used in CT imaging.[4] All of these factors mean that administration can be repeated as required.

Applications of ultrasound enhancement agents

The clinical applications of CEUS are increasing rapidly. Use of sono-graphic contrast agents is well established in echocardiography to improve endocardial border detection and is being developed for myo-cardial perfusion. CEUS can be used in the investigation of the liver and spleen, as well as imaging of the kidneys, pancreas, breast, prostate, testes and thyroid.[5] In conjunction with colourflow Doppler imaging, ultrasound contrast media may give valuable information in renal and hepatic perfusion studies and other vascular applications. A licence has recently been granted in the UK for the use of sonographic contrast agents in paediatric patients for vesico-ureteric reflux (VUR). It is important to note that not all agents have the same licensing indications in different countries and this should always be checked prior to use, as should the legal implications of sonographers administering contrast agents.

An inherent advantage of CEUS is the possibility of assessing the contrast enhancement patterns in real time with a substantially higher temporal resolution than other imaging modalities, without the need to predefine scan-time-points or to perform bolus tracking.

Microbubbles have clinical uses in many other applications where knowledge of the microcirculation is important. The macrocirculation can usually be assessed adequately using conventional Doppler, although there are a few important situations where the signal boost given by microbubbles is useful, for instance in transcranial Doppler evaluation of vasospasm after subarachnoid haemorrhage.

CEUS may have a role in abdominal trauma; injury to the liver, spleen and kidneys can be assessed rapidly and repeatedly if necessary. Its role here alongside dynamic CT remains to be evaluated. CEUS seems to be useful in the investigation of infarcts or ischaemia and other abnormal vascularities, especially in renal and splenic malignancies. Improved detection of the neovascularisation of ovarian carcinomas is promising. There may be similar benefits in the head and neck and in the skin, whereas the demonstration of the neovascularisation of atheromatous plaques and aggressive joint inflammation offers interesting potentials.

Unlike contrast agents for other modalities, microbubbles may be modified by the process used to image them. Bubble rupture under a burst of high-power ultrasound can release their content for targeted delivery of, for instance, chemotherapy. Future developments offer the prospect of molecular and cellular imaging, monitoring of drug therapy and drug and gene delivery.

Applications of CEUS are discussed with the corresponding images in:

- Chapter 2 'The upper abdominal organs' for liver haemangioma.
- Chapter 3 'The renal tract' for complex renal cyst.
- Chapter 7 'The female reproductive system' in the section on 'HyCoSy'.

FUSION IMAGING

Fusion imaging is the combination of two or more imaging modalities, so, in the case of ultrasound, it might be ultrasound with CT, MRI, or positron emission tomography (PET). Data from the images may be merged into a single composite image or the two images may be viewed side by side on one monitor. The combination of modalities optimises the best features of each, so the real-time visualisation plus the excellent spatial resolution of ultrasound may be combined with the higher contrast imaging of CT or MRI. Ultrasound technologies such as Doppler, elastography and CEUS may be applied, and the result can demonstrate both the anatomy and the function of an organ or lesion (**Figure 15.1**). Fusion imaging is therefore helpful in localising lesions for ultrasound-guided biopsy or therapeutic intervention.

Fusion imaging is particularly useful when lesions are isoechoic or difficult to locate on ultrasound, enabling the user to track the position of the transducer and locate the specific region of interest in an organ.

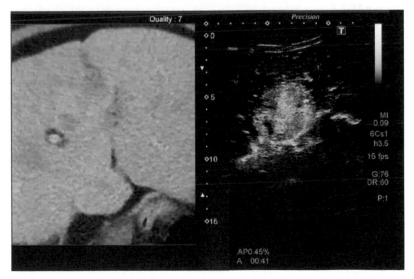

Figure 15.1 This combination of cross-sectional imaging with a contrast-enhanced ultrasound image demonstrates arterial enhancement of a liver metastasis.

Figure 15.2 shows the localisation of a tumour within the kidney. This was diagnosed as a renal cell carcinoma on biopsy.

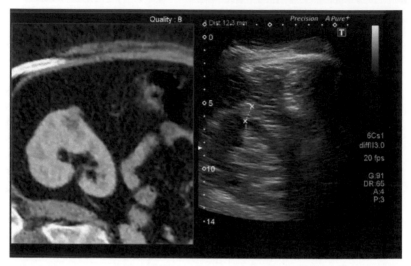

Figure 15.2 Fusion imaging, with the ultrasound image on the right, clearly identifies a renal lesion for biopsy.

Because ultrasound is a real-time imaging modality without the use of ionising radiation, it is often the preferred method of imaging to guide interventional procedures (**Figure 15.3**). Magnetic sensors are used to help position the probe.[6] Reusable trackers can be attached to the patient to compensate for breathing and other movements so as to ensure accurate positioning.

Fusion imaging has been found to improve short- and long-term outcomes for therapeutic lesion ablations, when compared with ultrasound guidance alone, particularly with the inclusion of CEUS.[7]

Applications for fusion imaging are increasing, as the technology develops. One such application is in assisting prostate biopsy. Prostate lesions can be difficult to identify on ultrasound but are clearly seen on MRI. Fusing the two images, as in **Figure 15.4**, enables real-time biopsy with increased accuracy.

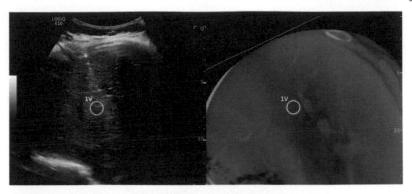

Figure 15.3 Targeting a lesion for biopsy using fusion imaging, with the ultrasound image on the left. The hyperechoic needle tip can be seen at the top left of the image. (Image reproduced with kind permission from GE.)

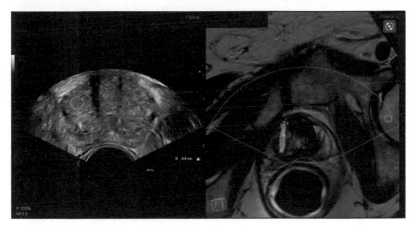

Figure 15.4 Fusion images of a transrectal ultrasound image of the prostate on the left and the corresponding magnetic resonance image on the right, to assist with the biopsy. (Image reproduced with kind permission from Esaote.)

343

ARTIFICIAL INTELLIGENCE (AI) IN ULTRASOUND

AI is the ability of technology to respond to a situation in a way that mimics human behaviour. AI has two subsets that are relevant for imaging: machine learning and deep learning (**Figure 15.5**).

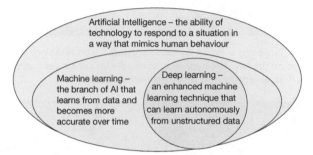

Figure 15.5 The interrelationship of artificial intelligence (AI), machine learning and deep learning. (Adapted from Drukker et al.[8])

Machine learning is the branch of AI that learns and becomes more accurate over time, developing algorithms based on data input. Machine learning and AI are used, for example, in websites and social media platforms to introduce targeted advertising, or to detect unusual activity such as spamming or illicit account access. Machine learning can be understood as a statistical method that gradually improves as it is exposed to more data, by extracting patterns from that data.[8] In terms of ultrasound images, machine learning needs images categorised by a range of factors such as normal or abnormal size, shape, outline, echotexture and vascularity.

Deep learning is an enhanced machine learning technique that differs from so-called 'smart' technology in that it is capable of learning autonomously from unstructured data, without human programming to do so. The data only need to be categorised as normal or abnormal or the anatomical structures to be labelled and, with huge training datasets, deep learning AI will start to recognise the defining features on its own. Once established, AI performs especially well in pattern recognition, and therefore it can be particularly helpful in medical imaging.[8] AI is already used widely in image analysis, for instance in the detection of intracerebral haemorrhage from CT images.[9]

Within ultrasound, there are immediately obvious advantages of computer assistance in accurate biometric measurements and in quality assessment. Deep learning can also be applied to more complex tasks in image acquisition and diagnostic analysis. These include detection and classification (What objects are within this image?), navigation (How do I move to acquire the optimal section?), segmentation (Where are the organ or lesion boundaries?) and registration (used to ensure an exact fit in image transfer to other modalities). These techniques show promise in enhancing CEUS, elastography and fusion imaging.[8,10]

Ultrasound images are subject to an inherent speckle artefact that sometimes prevents accurate observation of anatomical details. Although speckle is generally regarded as a hindrance, the generation of this artefact is related to the microstructure of the tissue and contains textural information that may prove useful for diagnostic purposes. Some subtle differences and repetition of patterns may be recognisable by AI where they are too nuanced for the human eye, resulting in achievement of the 'holy grail' of tissue characterisation, by extracting and recognising discriminative patterns of pathological conditions. AI has already achieved this in lung ultrasound, by the differentiation of COVID-19 lung appearances from other pathology that could not have been distinguished by humans alone, and enabling the rapid diagnosis of very large numbers of cases of COVID-19.[11]

In terms of biometry, AI can acquire, annotate, measure and archive standard sections, offering more accuracy and faster screening in vascular, gynaecological and fetal anomaly scanning. This may allow more time for analysis of additional scan planes, or for communication with patients[8] or to develop advanced clinical practice roles.

In vascular applications, AI is capable of plaque characterisation and automated measurement of intima-media thickness in carotid scanning. In surveillance of abdominal aortic aneurysms (AAAs), whether native or post endovascular aneurysm repair (EVAR), AI can provide the maximum anteroposterior (AP) diameter, plus other dimensions and partial volume of the aneurysm, while also indicating the centre line of the aneurysm.[12]

In obstetrics, AI can assist with the recognition of standard sections and with automatic measurements such as fetal head circumference, abdominal circumference and femur length. In gynaecological ultrasound, endometrial thickness can be detected and measured accurately, and ovarian cysts can be automatically classified using the IOTA (International Ovarian Tumor Analysis) criteria.[8] All of these applications can help to reduce intra- and inter-operator differences, to provide more consistency in diagnosis and follow-up of cases.

AI-assisted processes may be applied within numerous systems[10] as illustrated in **Figure 15.6**, which demonstrates potential options that could enhance the workflow of an ultrasound facility in terms of work-load management, scanning assistance and higher level functions.

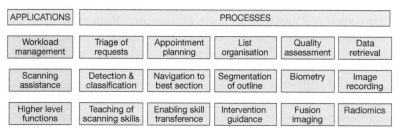

Figure 15.6 Some potential applications of AI within an ultrasound facility.

One of the criticisms of ultrasound as a modality is its operator dependence and AI assistance may help to eliminate some of these concerns. The AI functions of classification, navigation and segmentation also render great teaching possibilities, potentially reducing the time needed to acquire appropriate skills and competence. AI is the tutor that is always available, never tires and can tell the learner exactly where to move to get the best section and then point out the object borders (**Figures 15.7** and **15.8**).

Although AI has the capability to change the way that sonographers learn their physical scanning techniques and analyse their findings, it can only assist and not replace these processes. AI can, however, assist in the development of transferable skills to enable the transition from one area of practice to another, for instance in staff redeployment from screening programmes to lung examination during a coronavirus pandemic.

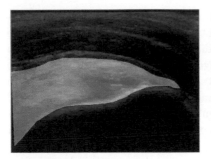

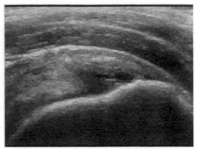

Figure 15.7 The segmentation mask detected by AI analysis overlaid on the image to highlight the region of interest. In this case, AI confirms the outline of the supraspinatus muscle.

Figure 15.8 The viewer is able to examine the supraspinatus muscle, once it has been positively identified in its full extent. The tendon is thickened and there is a hyperechoic area near the insertion into the greater tuberosity, suggesting a diagnosis of supraspinatus tendinosis.

Recent developments in deep learning techniques have produced an exciting new world for ultrasound. Images are usually acquired by the sonographer during a freehand scanning technique, and interpretation is best made in real time while the examination is being performed. Wireless probes can send data to 'the cloud' for AI processing, and the optimised image is then transmitted to the device screen (tablet or even smartphone), possibly even with a suggested diagnosis. The image appears to the operator as if it is 'real time' and the data are used for further deep learning. This generates ethical questions, and careful decisions will need to be made regarding who 'owns' the patient data that is fed back into systems to hone the accuracy of AI.

There can be a mistrust of AI, in part around the production of results without an explanation of the process, for instance in image interpretation. There are now attempts to develop 'explainable AI' (XAI) whereby some supporting evidence may be included in the results.[13] It is important that sufficient high-quality data are used for development and training of AI biometry systems to eliminate operator expectation bias from results.

As with any computing system, the output can only generate conclusions based on the original input, and it may be better to categorise appearances as urgent, for immediate review or routine, rather than providing a final diagnosis, as original data input is unlikely to have captured all potential pathologies. Although AI systems can perform some higher-level cognitive tasks, including differentiation of abnormal from normal appearances, and even provisional reporting of the conditions it 'knows', it is crucial that reporting sonographers have oversight to ensure accuracy and consistency.[14]

There are numerous other concerns over AI, particularly regarding safety. Regulatory bodies currently approve AI applications only if there are 'locked' parameters. This means that clinical applications use static models that can no longer adapt, so there is no increased machine learning or deep learning, and there can be no changes to the AI system over time.[15] It is also important that bias is not introduced into the AI system, so in health care a dataset should be derived from a diverse range of patients, representative of the populations being served.[16]

Promising developments include three-dimensional ultrasound and image-guided interventions for both diagnostic and therapeutic purposes, and the emerging field of radiomics, where AI is fused with clinical data, correlating an image pattern with laboratory findings. This has already shown promise in the classification of primary liver cancers.[17]

There is no doubt that AI will advance in diagnostic imaging as it has in other fields and change practice as it does so. The vast number of images, biometry and other data required to facilitate and direct machine learning in numerous applications will ensure not only a continuing role for the sonographer but also offer exciting opportunities for professional role expansion if AI development is embraced.

REFERENCES

1. Moon WK, Im JG, Noh DY, Han MC. Nonpalpable breast lesions: Evaluation with power Doppler US and a microbubble contrast agent – initial experience. *Radiology* 2000;**217**(1):240–246. doi: 10.1148/radiology.217.1.r00oc03240.

2. Delgado Oliva F, Arlandis Guzman S, Bonillo García M, Broseta Rico E, Boronat Tormo F. Diagnostic performance of power Doppler and ultrasound contrast agents in early imaging-based diagnosis of organ-confined prostate cancer: Is it possible to spare cores with contrast-guided biopsy? *European Journal of Radiology* 2016;**85**(10):1778–1785. doi: 10.1016/j.ejrad.2016.07.021.

3. Claudon M, Cosgrove D, Albrecht T, Bolondi L, Bosio M, Calliada F, et al. Guidelines and good clinical practice recommendations for contrast enhanced ultrasound (CEUS) – update 2008. *Ultraschall in der Medizin* 2008;**29**(1):28–44. doi: 10.1055/s-2007-963785.

4. Zanardo M, Doniselli FM, Esseridou A, Tritella S, Mattiuz C, Menicagli L, et al. Abdominal CT: A radiologist-driven adjustment of the dose of iodinated contrast agent approaches a calculation per lean body weight. *European Radiology Experimental* 2018;**2**(1):41. doi: 10.1186/s41747-018-0074-1

5. Cosgrove D. Ultrasound contrast agents: An overview. *European Journal of Radiology* 2006:**60**(3);324–330. doi: 10.1016/j.ejrad.2006.06.022.

6. Sandulescu DL, Dumitrescu D, Rogoveanu I, Saftoiu A. Hybrid ultrasound imaging techniques (fusion imaging). *World Journal of Gastroenterology* 2011;**17**(1):49–52. doi: 10.3748/wjg.v17.i1.49.

7. Ma QP, Xu EJ, Zeng QJ, Su ZZ, Tan L, Chen JX, et al. Intraprocedural computed tomography/magnetic resonance–contrast-enhanced ultrasound fusion imaging improved thermal ablation effect of hepatocellular carcinoma: Comparison with conventional ultrasound. *Hepatology Research* 2019;**49**(7):799–809. doi: 10.1111/hepr.13336.

8. Drukker L, Noble JA, Papageorghiou AT. Introduction to artificial intelligence in ultrasound imaging in obstetrics and gynecology. *Ultrasound in Obstetrics and Gynecology* 2020;**56**(4):498–505. doi: 10.1002/uog.22122.

9. Soun JE, Chow DS, Nagamine M, Takhtawala RS, Filippi CG, Yu W, et al. Artificial intelligence and acute stroke imaging. *American Journal of Neuroradiology* 2021;**42**(1):2–11. doi: 10.3174/ajnr.A6883.

10. Liu S, Wang Y, Yang X, Lei B, Liu L, Li XS, et al. Deep learning in medical ultrasound analysis: A review. *Engineering* 2019;**5**(2):261–275. doi: 1016/j.eng.2018.11.020.

11. Arntfield R, VanBerlo B, Alaifan T, Phelps N, White M, Chaudhary R, et al. Development of a deep learning classifier to accurately distinguish COVID-19 from look-a-like pathology on lung ultrasound. *medRxiv* 2020. doi: 10.1101/2020.10.13.20212258.

12. Philips. *Increased diagnostic confidence and improved patient experience: Philips abdominal aortic aneurysm (AAA) model.* Amsterdam: Philips, 2020:1–4. Available at: https://www.philips.com/c-dam/b2bhc/master/landing-pages/abdominal-aortic-aneurysm-model/philips-abdominal-aortic-aneurysm-model-leaflet.pdf.

13. Langlotz CP, Allen B, Erickson BJ, Kalpathy-Cramer J, Bigelow K, Cook TS, et al. A roadmap for foundational research on artificial intelligence in medical imaging: From the 2018 NIH/RSNA/ACR/The Academy Workshop. *Radiology* 2019;**291**(3):781–791. doi: 10.1148/radiol.2019190613.

14. Hardy M, Harvey H. Artificial intelligence in diagnostic imaging: Impact on the radiography profession. *British Journal of Radiology* 2020;**93**(1108):20190840. doi: 10.1259/bjr.20190840.

15. Babic B, Gerke S, Evgeniou T, Cohen IG. Algorithms on regulatory lockdown in medicine. *Science* 2019;**366**(6470):1202–1204. doi: 10.1126/science.aay9547.

16. Turpin R, Hoefer E, Lewelling J, Baird P. *Machine learning AI in medical devices: Adapting regulatory frameworks and standards to ensure safety and performance.* Arlington, VA: AAMI, BSI, 2020:1–24. Available at: https://www.ethos.co.im/wp-content/uploads/2020/11/MACHINE-LEARNING-AI-IN-MEDICAL-DEVICES-ADAPTING-REGULATORY-FRAMEWORKS-AND-STANDARDS-TO-ENSURE-SAFETY-AND-PERFORMANCE-2020-AAMI-and-BSI.pdf.

17. Peng Y, Lin P, Wu L, Wan D, Zhao Y, Liang L, et al. Ultrasound-based radiomics analysis for preoperatively predicting different histopathological subtypes of primary liver cancer. *Frontiers in Oncology* 2020;**10**:1646. doi: 10.3389/fonc.2020.01646.

INDEX

(Numbers in bold indicate figures)

A

abdomen
  spectral Doppler ultrasound 40
  trauma 323, **324–325**, 326,
    327–328
  upper 40–62
abdominal aortic aneurysm (AAA)
  212, **212**, 213–215, **216**
abdominal circumference (AC)
  181, 184, **184**, 189–190, **190**,
  191–193, 346
ABPI *see* ankle–brachial pressure
  index
ABUS *see* automated breast
  ultrasound
ABVS *see* automated breast volume
  scanning
Achilles tendon 310, **311**
  normal **312**
  tear **312**
acoustic enhancement 6
acoustic shadowing **7**
acquired immune deficiency
  syndrome (AIDS) 58
acromioclavicular (AC) joint 280,
  282, **284**
acute appendicitis 113, **114**, 115
adenocarcinoma, pancreatic 46, **47**
adenomyosis, uterus 146, 148, **149**
ADNEX 151
adnexae 145–146, 151, 171, 180
adrenal glands 135–139
  adenoma 130, 137, **137**
  metastatic mass **139**
  phaeochromocytoma **138**
  position **136**

power Doppler ultrasound
  137–138
adrenocortical carcinoma 138
allergy 27
anaesthetics 314–317
aneurysm
  aorta 212, **212**, 213–215, 216
  artificial intelligence 345
  colourflow Doppler ultrasound
    216
  endovascular repair (EVAR)
    345
angiomyolipoma, kidney 74, **74**
angioplasty, intravascular
  ultrasound 252–254
anisotropy
  ankle 308
  biceps tendon **282**, 283
  elbow 287
  wrist 293
ankle 308–313
  Achilles tendon 310, **311**
  colourflow Doppler ultrasound
    308
  power Doppler ultrasound 308
ankle–brachial pressure index
  (ABPI) 222–223, **225**, 231
annular array imaging **119**
anterior tibial artery **224**
aorta 212–216
  aneurysm 212, **212**, 213–215,
    216
  normal **215**
aortic valve 244–245, **246–247**
appendicitis, acute 113, **114**, 115
arteriovenous malformations 232
artificial intelligence 344, **344**,
  345–346, **346–347**, 347–348
assisted reproduction 157–160

atherosclerosis 226
    artery 253, **254**
automated breast ultrasound
    (ABUS) 206
automated breast volume scanning
    (ABVS) 206
axillary vein 237, **238–239**
    colourflow Doppler ultrasound
        238

B
B mode 7–8, **8**, 9, 13
Baker's cyst, knee 304, 307, **307**
benign colloid nodule, thyroid
    gland 133, **134**
benign prostatic hypertrophy
    (BPH) 83
biceps muscle 280, 287
biceps tendon 281–282, **282–283**,
    285
    anisotropy **282**
bile duct 48
    common (CBD) 46, **46**, 54, **54**,
        119
    intrahepatic 46
    stone **119**
    tumour 41
biliary tree 41, 43, 46, 54
    normal **119**
bladder 78–83
    calculi 82, **82**, 83
    colourflow Doppler ultrasound
        81
    debris **82**
    fetal 177, 185, **185**
    normal **80, 81**
    polyps 83
    pregnancy 171
    thickened wall **81**
    TRUS 88–89
    urothelial carcinoma **83**

blood vessels, intravascular
    ultrasound 252–254
Bosniak classification 73
bowel 113–116, 123, **123**
    contrast-enhanced ultrasound
        (CEUS) 113
    Crohn's disease **115**, 116
    intussusception **115**
    obstruction 42
BPH *see* benign prostatic
    hypertrophy
brachial artery 224, 230
brachial vein 237
    thrombosis **238**
brachialis muscle 285, 287
brain
    extracranial arteries 217–223
    neonatal 272–277, **275–277**
breast 198–208
    automated-motion transducer
        206
    carcinoma 202, **202**, **205**, 208,
        208
    contrast-enhanced ultrasound
        (CEUS) 198–203
    cyst **202**
    fibroadenoma 201–202, **205**
    invasive ductal carcinoma **202**,
        208
    mass **203**
    normal **201**
    power Doppler ultrasound 198,
        202–203, **203**
brightness modulated mode *see*
    B mode
bursitis
    elbow 285, 288
    foot 308
    patellar tendon 306, **306**
    subacromial **316–317**
    trochanteric 315

C

calculi
  bladder 82, **82**, 83
  renal 71, **71**, 76
  submandibular gland 110, **111**
calf veins 234, **234**
cancer antigen 125 (CA125) 143
carcinoma
  adrenocortical 138
  breast 202, **202**, **205**, 208, **208**
  colon **116**
  medullary 202
  ovarian 143, 340
  renal cell 342
  testicular 94
  urothelial 82, 83, **83**
cardiac angiography, intravascular
  ultrasound 252–254
cardiac probes 239 240, **241–243**,
  244–245, 249, **249**
cardiac tamponade 323, **324–325**
carotid artery 10, 217–218,
  218–221, 219
  common (CCA) **131**, 218–221,
    219–220
  external (ECA) 218–219
  internal (ICA) 218–219, 221
  normal **219–220**
  stenosis **221**
carpal tunnel 289, 291, **291–292**,
  292–293, **293**
cavernosal artery 103
cell-free non-invasive prenatal
  testing (cfNIPT) 177
cerebral artery 193
CEUS see contrast-enhanced
  ultrasound
CFA see common femoral artery
CFV see common femoral vein
chorionic villus sampling (CVS)
  166, 175, 177

chronic pancreatitis **47**
ciliary body muscle 270
CMUT (capacitive micromachined
  ultrasonic transducer) array 12
colon
  carcinoma **116**
  tumour 120, **120**
colourflow Doppler ultrasound 9,
  9, 10, **10**, 19
common bile duct (CBD) 46, **46**,
  54, **54**, 119
common carotid artery (CCA)
    131, 218–221, **219–220**
  colourflow Doppler ultrasound
    219, **220–221**
  duplex imaging **220**
  spectral Doppler ultrasound
    218–219, **220**
  triplex imaging 219, **220**
common duct 54, **54–55**
common extensor tendon 286,
  288, **288**, 315
common femoral artery (CFA)
    224, **227–229**, 228, 235, **236**
  colourflow Doppler ultrasound
    228
  duplex imaging **229**
common femoral vein (CFV) 228,
    228, 232, 235, **235–236**
  colourflow Doppler ultrasound
    235
  spectral Doppler ultrasound
    235
common flexor tendon 286, 288,
  288
common hepatic duct (CHD) 54,
  54, 119
common iliac artery **224**
communication 22, 26, 27, 32,
  122, 171, 273, 304, 211, 331,
  345

ASCKS framework, obstetric ultrasound **24**, 25
clinical report writing 31–34
delivering unexpected findings 23
computed tomography 2, **6**
liver **52**
Computerized Imaging Reference Systems (CIRS) **18**
concave probes 207
continuous wave (CW) ultrasound 11, 223–226, 244
contraception, intrauterine system (IUS) 149, **150**
contrast agents 338, 339
contrast-enhanced ultrasound (CEUS) 338–340
artificial intelligence 345
bowel 113
breast 198–203
fusion imaging 341–342
HyCoSy 152–156
liver 50–51, **52**
prostate 83
renal 73–74, **73**
coronary artery 252–253, **254**
COVID-19, lung 258, 263, **263**, 345
Crohn's disease, bowel **115**
crown–rump length (CRL) 168, 176–177, **178**
cubital tunnel 286
curvilinear probes 11, 43, 48, **49**, 58, 69, **69**, 79, **79**, 113, **114**, 142, **142**, 180
cyst
Baker's 304, 307, **307**
epidermoid 99, **99**
epididymal 96, **97**
haemorrhagic **151**
ovarian 80, 150, **150–151**, 151, 153, 157, 346
polycystic kidney 68, 73, **73**, 74
renal 72, **72–73**, 73
rete testis **96**
splenic 61, **62**
testicular **98**

D
decontamination, probes 28, 273
deep femoral artery **224**
deep vein thrombosis (DVT) 232, 237, **238**
colourflow Doppler ultrasound 232–234, 237, 238
duplex imaging 232, **238**
deltoid muscle 283, **317**
developmental dysplasia of the hip (DDH) 294–295, **298**, 299–300, **301**
diaphragm
congenital hernia 186
pleural effusion **61**, 259, **259**, 260, **264**
digital artery 230
distal biceps tendon 287, **287**
Doppler 8–11
colourflow 9–10
continuous wave (CW) 11, 223–226, 244
power 10
spectral 9
dorsalis pedis artery **224**
Down's syndrome 175–177
duplex imaging 9
carotid arteries 217–223
common femoral artery (CFA) **229**
deep vein thrombosis 232, **238**
heart 245
liver **51**

mitral valve **247**
short saphenous vein 234, **234**
subclavian artery **231**
vertebral arteries **222**
dysplasia 273
paediatric hip 294–295, **297**, **298**, 299–300, 301
skeletal 184, 186
see also Graf classification

E
echocardiography, heart 239–248
ectopic pregnancy 156, 169, 171, 174, **174**
Edwards' syndrome 175–177, 186
eFAST (extended focused assessment with sonography in trauma) 322
elastography, breast 204–205
elbow 285–288
colourflow Doppler ultrasound 285
power Doppler ultrasound 285
electrocardiogram (ECG) 239, 244
endocavitary probes 28, 88
endometrioma, ovary 160, **160**
endometrium **144**, 145–148, **147**, 152
polyps 147, **147**, 157, 159
endoprobes 253
endoscopic retrograde cholangio-pancreatography (ERCP) 330
endoscopic ultrasound (EUS)
gastrointestinal tract 117–121
portal vein **119**
endovascular aneurysm repair (EVAR) 345
epidermoid cyst 99, **99**
epididymis, cyst 96, **97**
epididymitis 93, **97**

colourflow Doppler ultrasound 97, **97**
epigastric region 43, **44–46**, 54
erectile dysfunction (ED) 103
ergonomics **30–31**
EUS *see* endoscopic ultrasound
external carotid artery (ECA) 218–219
external iliac artery **224**
extracranial arteries 217–223
colourflow Doppler ultrasound 217
spectral Doppler ultrasound 217
extracranial imaging *see* duplex imaging
extraocular muscle 271
extrarenal pelvis 71, **72**
eye 268–272
colourflow Doppler ultrasound 270
foreign body **272**
normal **270**
retinal detachment **271**

F
facial artery 110, **111**
fallopian tubes 152
blocked 156
hysterosalpingo-contrast sonography (HyCoSy) 154, **155–156**, 156
rupture 174
FAST (focused assessment with sonography in trauma) 322–329
femoral artery 226, **227–229**
common (CFA) **224**, **227–229**, 228, 235, **236**
deep **224**
spectral Doppler ultrasound 227, **229**
superficial **224**

triphasic flow **229**
femoral vein, common (CFV) 228, **228**, 232, 235, **235–236**
femur length (FL), fetus 181, 184, 189, **191**, 193
fertility 152–156
fetal growth restriction (FGR) 166, 188, 191–193
fetus
  first trimester 176
  second trimester 179, 181, 184, 185, 187
  third trimester 188–192
  abdominal circumference (AC) 181, 184, **184**, 189–190, **190**, 191–193, 346
  bladder 177, 185, **185**
  calliper placement **182–184**
  crown–rump length (CRL) 168, 176–177, **178**
  femur length (FL) 181, 184, 189, **191**, 193
  growth restriction 166, 188, 191–193
  head circumference (HC) 168, 176, 179, 181, **182**, 189, **190**, 191–193
  heart **186**
  lips **183**
  nasal tip **183**
  nuchal fold **183**
  nuchal translucency 176–177
  spine **185**
  transcerebellar diameter (TCD) 182, **183**
fibroadenoma, breast 201–202, **205**
fibroids 149, 153, 157, 159
  endometrium 148
  myometrium 147–148
  uterus 146, **148**

fibular ligaments 309
flexor carpi radialis 292, **292–293**
flexor pollicis longus 291–292, **292–293**
flexor retinaculum 291–292, **292**, 293
focal nodular hyperplasia (FNH) 34
focused assessment with sonography in trauma *see* FAST
follicle tracking 157, 159, **159–160**
foot 308–313
  Morton's neuroma 308, 311, **311**, 313, **313**
foreign body, eye **272**
frequency 2–3, 8–9, 11–12, **12**, 13
fusion imaging 341–343
  contrast-enhanced ultrasound (CEUS) 341–342

G
gallbladder 53–55
gallstones **7**, **53**
gastrocnemius muscle 310
gastroduodenal artery **46**
gastrointestinal tract (GI), adult 112–121
  colourflow Doppler ultrasound 118
  intussusception **115**
  polyps 118
gastrointestinal tract (GI), neonate 121–123
gestation sac, uterus **172–173**
glomerular filtration rate, estimated (eGFR) 68
goitre, multinodular 132, **132**
Graf classification 295–303
  type 1 hip **299**, 300, **301**
  type 2a hip 300, **301**
  type 2b hip 300

type 2c hip 300
type 3 hip 300
type 4 hip 300, **302**
type D hip 300
Graf technique 295, **295,**
296–299
Graves' disease, thyroid gland **132**
gynaecology 142–152

H
haemangioma, liver **53**
haematuria 82, 83
haemoperitoneum 323
haemorrhage, intraventricular
(IVH) 277, **277**
haemorrhagic cyst **151**
hand 289–293
Hashimoto's thyroiditis **132**
head
anatomy **182**
neonate 273–274, **274**
transcerebellar diameter (TCD)
182, **183**
head circumference (HC) 168,
176, 179, 181, **182,** 189, **190,**
191–193
heart
3D reconstruction **251**
colourflow Doppler ultrasound
244–245, 248, 250
duplex imaging 245
echocardiography 239–248,
245, 247
muscle 42
pericardial fluid **328**
spectral Doppler ultrasound
244
transoesophageal
echocardiography (TOE)
249–251, **251**
hepatic artery 54, **119**

hepatic duct, common (CHD) 54,
54, 119
hepatic veins 50, 57
stent 333
triphasic flow **51**
hepatomegaly **50**
high-frequency probes 83, 316
high-intensity focused ultrasound
(HIFU) 331
hip, infant 293–303
hormone fluctuations, menstrual
cycle **144**
human chorionic gonadotrophin
(hCG) 100, 143, 169
human immunodeficiency virus
(HIV) 58
HyCoSy *see* hysterosalpingo-
contrast sonography
hydrocele, testis **98**
hydronephrosis, kidney **75**
hysterosalpingo-contrast
sonography (HyCoSy) 152–156
contrast-enhanced ultrasound
(CEUS) 152–156
fallopian tubes 154, **155–156,**
156
peritoneum 153, 156, **156**
uterus **155**

I
iliac artery 213
common **224**
external **224**
inferior vena cava (IVC) **45,** 50,
51, 74, 189, 214
infertility
female 152–160
male (erectile dysfunction)
103–105
infraspinatus muscle 280, **281,**
282

infraspinatus tendon **284**
internal carotid artery (ICA)
218–219, 221
International Ovarian Tumor
Analysis (IOTA) 32, 346
interventions 328–334, **334**
interventional procedures, MSK
314–317
interventional ultrasound
330–334
shoulder **316–317**
intrauterine system (IUS),
contraception 149, **150**
intravascular ultrasound (IVUS)
252–254
intraventricular haemorrhage
(IVH) 277, **277**
intussusception, abdomen **115**

J
jugular vein 10, 219, **220**, 237
normal **220**

K
kidneys 68–77
angiomyolipoma **74**
duplex **72**
ectopic 72
extrarenal pelvis **72**
hydronephrosis **75**
nephrocalcinosis **76**
normal **70**
polycystic 68, 73, **73**, 74
power Doppler ultrasound 74,
77
solid lesion **74**
urinary tract infection **76**
knee 303–307
Baker's cyst **307**

L
Legge–Calve–Perthes disease
(LCPD) **294**
ligaments, medial collateral **307**
limbs
colourflow Doppler ultrasound
226–227, 230–231
lower segmental pressure **224**
peripheral arteries 223–231
peripheral veins 232–239
spectral Doppler ultrasound
226, 230, 233
Lister's tubercle **292**
liver
biopsy **334**
cirrhosis **57**
common bile duct (CBD) 46,
46, 54, **54**, 119
common duct **54–55**
common hepatic duct (CHD)
54, **54**, 119
contrast-enhanced ultrasound
(CEUS) 50–51, **52**
cyst, anechoic **7**
duplex imaging **51**
haemangioma **53**
hepatomegaly **50**
metastasis **341**
metastatic disease **52**
normal 50–51
porta hepatis **55**
long saphenous vein (LSV) 228,
228, **236**
low-frequency probes 225
lower urinary tract symptoms
(LUTS) 83
lungs 258–264
COVID-19 **263**
M mode 261, **261**
normal **261–262**
pleural effusion **264**

lymph nodes **134**
lymphoma, spleen **62**
   colourflow Doppler ultrasound
     62

M
M mode 7–8, **8**, 26
   echocardiography 239
   fetal heart 171
   lung 261, **261**
   mitral valve 244, 246, **246**, 247,
     247
magnetic resonance
   cholangiopancreatography
   (MRCP) 43
magnetic resonance imaging (MRI)
   2, **6**, **52**
mass, breast **203**
mechanical index (MI) 14
medial cerebral artery **275**
medial collateral ligament **307**
mediastinum testis 96, **96**
medullary carcinoma 202
menstrual cycle **144**, 145–148, 152
mesenteric artery, superior 43,
   44–45, 214, **215**
metastasis
   adrenal gland **139**
   liver **52**, **341**
microlithiasis, testis **101**
mitral valve **186**, 244, **246–248**,
   248, **251**
   duplex imaging **247**
   leaflets **247**
   M mode 244, 246, **246**, 247,
     247
   spectral Doppler ultrasound
     248
   triplex imaging **248**
Morton's neuroma 308, 311, **311**,
   313, **313**

movement modulated mode *see*
   M mode
multinodular goitre 132, **132**
muscle
   biceps 280, 287
   bipennate 287
   brachialis 285, 287
   ciliary body 270
   deltoid 283, **317**
   extraocular 271
   gastrocnemius 310
   heart 42
   hypertrophy 230
   infraspinatus 280, **281**, 282
   mylohyoid 108
   pectoralis **201**
   rotator cuff 280, **281**
   soleus 310
   strap 130, **131**
   subscapularis 280
   supraspinatus 280, **347**
   tendon junction 291
   teres minor 280, **281**, 282
   triceps 286
mylohyoid muscle 108

N
Neck 128–134
necrotising enterocolitis (NEC),
   neonatal bowel 113, 121, **123**
neonates
   bowel, necrotising enterocolitis
     123
   brain 272–277, **275–277**
   gut, normal **123**
   head 273–274, **274**
   intraventricular haemorrhage
     277
nephrocalcinosis 76
Newborn and Infant Physical
   Examination (NIPE) 20

nodule, thyroid gland 128, 132,
  132–133, 133, **134**
nuchal fold (NF), fetus 182, **183**
nuchal translucency 175–176, **178**

O
obstetric ultrasound 166–196
  ASCKS framework **24**
  bladder 171
  ectopic 156, 169, 171, 174, **174**
  first trimester 175–178, **178**,
    179
  growth graph **191**
  normal amniotic fluid **192**
  normal umbilical artery **193**
  nuchal translucency **178**
  second trimester 179–182, **182**,
    183–187
  third trimester **169**, 188–193
    abdomen **190**
    femur **191**
    head **190**
  transvaginal scan (TVS)
    169–172, **172**, 174, 188
  twins 173, **173**, 181
occlusive arterial disease 224
omental biopsy 329, 333, **334**
optical coherence tomography
  (OCT) 252
ovarian hyperstimulation
  syndrome (OHSS) 157
ovaries
  carcinoma 143, 340
  cyst **150–151**
  endometrioma 160, **160**
  follicle tracking **160**
  haemorrhagic cyst **151**
  malignancy **329**
  menstrual cycle **144**
  polycystic 153, 157
  tumour **152**

P
paediatric hip dysplasia 294–295,
  295–298, 296–300, **300–302**,
  301–303
pancreas 46, **46**, 47, 54, **54**,
  117–118, 339
  pseudocyst drainage **120**
pancreatic adenocarcinoma 46, **47**
pancreatic duct (PD) 42, 45–46,
  46–47, 54
pancreatitis 42, 45–46
  acute 42, 45
  chronic **47**
  pancreatic pseudocyst **46**
parotid gland 108, 110
  colourflow Doppler ultrasound
    110
  tumour **112**
Patau's syndrome 175–177, 186
patella 304–305
patellar tendon 303, **304**,
    305–306
  bursitis **306**
  normal **306**
patient preparation 21–26
Pavlik harness 301, **302**
peak systolic velocity (PSV) 70,
  193, 220–222, 227–228
pectoralis muscle **201**
pelvi-ureteric junction (PUJ),
  obstruction 75–76
pelvis
  FAST (focused assessment
    with sonography in trauma)
    322–323, **329**
  gynaecology 142–143, 145, 160
  obstetrics 170–171, 174, 176,
    180
  renal 68–69, 71–72, 75, 77
penis 103–105
  arteriovenous fistula 104, **104**

colourflow Doppler ultrasound 105, **105**
priapism 104, **105**
post-priapism infarction **105**
spectral Doppler ultrasound 104, **104**
triplex imaging **104**
percutaneous umbilical blood sampling (PUBS) 179
pericardium 322–325, 328, **328**
peripheral arteries
  lower limb 223–229
  upper limb 230–231
peripheral veins
  lower limb 232–236
  upper limb 237–239
phaeochromocytoma, adrenal gland 138, **138**
phased array probes 239
pinch grip, ergonomics 30, **31**
pleural effusion, diaphragm **61**, 259, **259**, 260, **264**
PMUT (piezoelectric micromachined ultrasonic transducer) array 12
polycystic ovaries 153, 157
polyps
  bladder 83
  endometrium 147, **147**, 157, 159
  gastrointestinal 118
  gynaecology 148
popliteal artery **224**, 226
popliteal vein 232
porta hepatis, liver 41, 54, 55
portal hypertension 56, 58, 333
portal vein 40, 55, **55**, 56, **56**, 57, **57**
  colourflow Doppler ultrasound 55–56, **56**, 57, 333
  endoscopic ultrasound **119**
  liver cirrhosis **57**

patency **333**
spectral Doppler ultrasound 55–57, **56**
stent 333
transjugular intrahepatic portosystemic shunt **57**
positron emission tomography (PET) 341
posterior acoustic enhancement **6**
posterior tibial artery **224**
pouch of Douglas 325, **325–326**, 326
power Doppler ultrasound 10, **10**, 19
pregnancy *see* obstetric ultrasound
priapism, penis 104, **105**
probes 3–4, 11–13, **11**
  concave 207
  curvilinear **11**, 43, 48, **49**, 58, 69, **69**, 79, **79**, 113, **114**, 142, **142**, 180
  damaged 16–17, **16**
  decontamination 28, 273
  endocavitary 28, 88
  endoprobe 253
  high-frequency 83, 316
  low-frequency 225
  phased array 239
  transabdominal 145, 170–171, 176, 180–181, 190
  transoesophageal 249, **249**
  transrectal 89–90
  transvaginal 23, 142, **142**, 143, 145, 153, 154, 158
  wireless 369
prostate gland 88–92
  biopsy 92, **343**
  contrast-enhanced ultrasound (CEUS) 152–156
  normal 90
  prostatic mass 91

transabdominal image **88**
prostate-specific antigen (PSA)
83, 88–89
pseudocyst drainage, pancreas **120**
pulmonary artery **264**
pulsed wave ultrasound 223, 244

R
radial artery 230
recto-uterine pouch **325–326**
renal artery 68, 70, 77, 213–214
colourflow Doppler ultrasound
70
spectral Doppler ultrasound 70
stenosis (RAS) 70
renal calculi 71, **71**, 76
colourflow Doppler ultrasound
71
twinkle artefact 71
renal cell carcinoma (RCC) 74,
342, **342**
colourflow Doppler ultrasound
74
renal cyst 72, **72–73**, 73
contrast-enhanced ultrasound
(CEUS) 73–74, **73**
renal vein 74
thrombosis 74
rete testis 96, 99
retina **270**, 271
detached 268, 271, **271**
retroperitoneum 46
retroverted uterus 146, **147**
reverberation 71, **71**
rotator cuff 280–284

S
safety 26–34
salivary glands 108–112
colourflow Doppler ultrasound
110–111, 112

power Doppler ultrasound **112**,
113
see also submandibular gland
saphenofemoral junction (SFJ)
235, **236**
saphenous vein **228**
short (SSV) 233, **234**
long (LSV) 228, **228**, **236**
scrotum 92–102
internal structures **93**
normal **95**
segmental pressure, lower limb
224
seminoma, testis 100, **100**
shear wave elastography (SWE)
204
short saphenous vein (SSV) 233,
234
duplex imaging 234, **234**
shoulder 280–284
colourflow Doppler ultrasound
316
ergonomics **30–31**
interventions **316–317**
power Doppler ultrasound 316
soleus muscle 310
SonoElastography *see* elastography
spectral Doppler ultrasound 9, **9**,
19
spermatic tubules *see* rete testis
sphygmomanometer 225, **225**
spina bifida 185–186
spleen 61–62
blunt trauma **61**
cyst 61, **62**
lymphoma **62**
normal **60**
power Doppler ultrasound 62
right lateral decubitus position
59
splenomegaly **60**

splenunculus **60**
splenic vein (SV) 43, **45**
splenomegaly **60**
splenunculus **60**
spongiform pattern nodule **133**
SSV *see* short saphenous vein
steroid injections 314–317
stone
    bladder 68
    common bile duct **119**
    gallstone **7**, 42, 46, 53, **53**, 54,
        117, 120
    kidney 71
    mandible 108
    pancreas 47
    penis 103
strap muscle 130, **131**
subacromial bursitis 283, 315,
    316–317, 317
subclavian artery 222, 230,
    230–231, 231
    colourflow Doppler ultrasound
        231, **231**
    duplex imaging **231**
    normal **231**
    spectral Doppler ultrasound
        230
subclavian steal syndrome 222
subclavian vein 231, 237
submandibular gland
    calculi 110, **111**
    colourflow Doppler ultrasound
        111
    normal **111**
subscapularis muscle 280
subscapularis tendon 281, 283,
    283
superficial femoral artery **224**
superior mesenteric artery (SMA)
    43, **44–45**, 214, **215**
supraspinatus muscle 280, **347**

supraspinatus tendon 281, 283,
    284
    tendinosis 347

T
tarsal tunnel 308
tendon
    biceps **282–283**
    colourflow Doppler ultrasound
        289
    common extensor **288**
    common flexor **288**
    infraspinatus **284**
    patellar **306**
    subscapularis **283**
    supraspinatus **281**, **284**
teres minor
    muscle 280, **281**, 282
testes 92–102
    carcinoma 94
    colourflow Doppler ultrasound
        102
    cyst 98
    hydrocele 98
    microlithiasis **101**
    normal 92–94, **95**
    power Doppler ultrasound 94,
        96
    seminoma **100**
    spectral Doppler ultrasound 94
    undescended 93, 101
    varicocele **101–102**
testicular artery **93**
testicular vasculature, normal **96**
TGC *see* time gain compensation
    controls
therapeutic lesion ablations 342,
    343
thermal index (TI) 14
thoracic outlet syndrome 230
thrombosis

deep vein (DVT) 232, 237, **238**
power Doppler ultrasound 237
renal vein 74, 77
right brachial vein 237, **238**
thyroid gland 128–134
  benign colloid nodule **134**
  colourflow Doppler ultrasound
    130
  diffuse changes **132**
  Graves' disease **132**
  Hashimoto's thyroiditis **132**
  multinodular goitre **132**
  nodule **133**
  normal **131**
  spongiform pattern nodule **133**
tibial artery, posterior **224**
time gain compensation (TGC)
  13–14, **14**, 82
transabdominal probes 145,
  170–171, 176, 180–181, 190
transcerebellar diameter (TCD)
  182, **183**
transducer decontamination **28**
transient ischaemic attack (TIA)
  217
transitional cell carcinoma (TCC)
  see urothelial carcinoma
transjugular intrahepatic
  portosystemic shunt (TIPSS)
  55, 57, **57**, 333
transoesophageal echocardiography
  (TOE) 249–251, **249**
transrectal ultrasound (TRUS) 83,
  343
  prostate gland 88–92
transvaginal probe 89, 142, **142**,
  143, 153–154, 158
transvaginal scan (TVS) 23, 143
  M mode 171
  ovarian cyst **151**
  ovarian tumour **152**

pregnancy 166, 169–172, **172**,
  174, 188
uterus 146, **146–147**, **149–150**
trauma 322–329
triceps muscle 286
triceps tendon 285, 287, **287**
triphasic flow
  femoral artery **229**
  hepatic veins **51**
triplex imaging
  arteriovenous (AV) fistula **104**
  carotid artery 219, **220**
  common femoral vein 235, **235**
  mitral valve **248**
  vertebral artery 222
trochanteric bursitis 315
tumour
  colon **120**
  kidney **74**
  ovary **152**
  parotid gland **112**
  *see also individual types of
    tumours*
twin pregnancy 173, **173**, 181

U
ulnar artery 230
ultrasound
  colourflow *see* colourflow
    Doppler ultrasound
  continuous wave (CW) 11,
    223–226, 244
  contrast-enhanced (CEUS) *see*
    contrast-enhanced ultrasound
  Doppler *see* Doppler ultrasound
  endoscopic (EUS) 117–121
  high-intensity focused
    ultrasound (HIFU) 331
  probes *see* probes
  power *see* power Doppler
    ultrasound

pulsed wave 223, 244
spectral *see* spectral Doppler
 ultrasound
umbilical artery 9, 9, 193, **193**
 spectral Doppler ultrasound
 193
umbilical vein **184**, 190
ureter
 spectral Doppler ultrasound 76
urinary bladder 78–83
urinary tract, lower symptoms
 (LUTS) 83
urinary tract infection (UTI)
 kidney 75, 76, **76**
 prostate 97
urothelial carcinoma 82, 83, **83**
uteropelvic junction (UPJ) 75
uterus
 adenomyosis 146, 148, **149**
 anteverted 146, **146**, 147, 171
 colourflow Doppler ultrasound
 10, 146, 148–149
 congenital abnormalities
 158–159
 fibroids 146, **148**
 follicle tracking **159–160**
 gestation sac **172–173**
 hysterosalpingo-contrast
 sonography (HyCoSy) **155**
 normal 149, **150**
 power Doppler ultrasound **10**,
 146

retroverted **147**
transvaginal scan (TVS) 146,
 146–147, **149–150**
two cavities **158–159**

V
varicocele, testis **101–102**, 102
varicose veins 232–234
vena cava, inferior (IVC) **45**, 50,
 51, 74, 189, 214
ventricular atrium (VA) 181, **182**
vertebral artery 217–218, 222,
 222–223, 231
 colourflow Doppler ultrasound
 218, 222
 duplex imaging **222**
 spectral Doppler ultrasound
 222, **223**
 triplex imaging 222
vesico-ureteric reflux (VUR) 340
volume scanning, breast 206–208

W
whole breast ultrasound (WBUS)
 see volume scanning
wireless probes 369
work-related musculoskeletal
 disorders (WRMSDs) 27,
 29–31
wrist 289–293
 power Doppler ultrasound 289

T - #0071 - 111024 - C388 - 198/129/18 [20] - CB - 9780367775087 - Gloss Lamination